Kyriakos Anastasiadis · Chandi Ratnatunga (Eds.)

The Thymus Gland

Kyriakos Anastasiadis · Chandi Ratnatunga (Eds.)

The Thymus Gland

Diagnosis and Surgical Management

With 61 Figures and 20 Tables

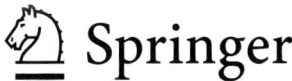

Springer

Kyriakos Anastasiadis
Aristotle University of Thessaloniki
Cardiothoracic Department
AHEPA Hospital
Thessaloniki
Greece
E-mail: anastasiadisk@hotmail.com

Chandi Ratnatunga
Department of Cardiothoracic Surgery
John Radcliffe Hospital
Oxford OX3 9DU
United Kingdom
E-mail: alison.horner@orh.nhs.uk

ISBN   978-3-540-33425-5   Springer Berlin Heidelberg New York

Library of Congress Control Number: 2006934461

Springer-Verlag is a part of Springer Science+Business Media
springer.com

© Springer-Verlag Berlin Heidelberg 2007

Editor: Gabriele M. Schröder, Heidelberg, Germany
Desk Editor: Stephanie Benko, Heidelberg, Germany
Cover design: Frido Steinen-Broo, eStudio Calamar, Spain
Typesetting and Production: LE-TeX Jelonek, Schmidt & Vöckler GbR, Leipzig, Germany

Printed on acid-free paper   24/3180/YL   5 4 3 2 1 0

Preface

"Εν οίδα ότι ουδέν οίδα…"

This saying by the Greek philosopher Socrates means: "What I know is that I know nothing", which is fitting to the thymus gland because the more you deal with it the more you believe you know very little about it.

Our aim was to write a book on the thymus gland that would familiarize the reader with the gland and provide, as a readily accessible guide, the background of knowledge necessary to follow the updates and controversies in the field. Although we tried to clear up various controversies about the thymus, there are still many left unsolved. That is why we believe readers will agree with the above-mentioned quote by Socrates.

We want to thank the coauthors for their contribution to the manuscript, as well as our secretaries, Mrs. Alison Horner and Mrs. Athina Tzili, for their various contributions. We also want to thank Mrs. Stephanie Benko, the book's Springer supervisor, for her patience and for the excellent job she did throughout the project.

K. Anastasiadis
C. Ratnatunga

Contents

List of Contributors

Kyriakos Anastasiadis
Aristotle University of Thessaloniki
Cardiothoracic Department
AHEPA Hospital
Thessaloniki
Greece
E-mail: anastasiadisk@hotmail.com

Kirsty Anderson
Radiology Department
Churchill Hospital
Old Road
Oxford OX3 9LJ
United Kingdom
E-mail: kirsty@kirstyanderson.com

Nick Bates
Radiology Department
Churchill Hospital
Old Road
Oxford OX3 9LJ
United Kingdom
E-mail: nick.bates@orh.nhs.uk

Penny Bradbury
Department of Medical Oncology
Princess Margaret Hospital
610 University Avenue
Toronto, Ontario M5G 2M9
Canada
E-mail: Penny.Bradbury@uhn.on.ca

Camilla Buckley
Department of Neurology
Radcliffe Infirmary
Woodstock Road
Oxford OX2 6HE
United Kingdom
E-mail: camilla.buckley@clinical-neurology.oxford.ac.uk

Colin Clelland
Department of Pathology Level 1
John Radcliffe Hospital
Oxford OX3 9DU
United Kingdom
E-mail: colin.clelland@orh.nhs.uk

Fergus Gleeson
Radiology Department
Churchill Hospital
Old Road
Oxford OX3 9LJ
United Kingdom
E-mail: fergus.gleeson@nds.ox.ac.uk

Chandi Ratnatunga
Department of Cardiothoracic Surgery Level 1
John Radcliffe Hospital
Oxford OX3 9DU
United Kingdom
E-mail: alison.horner@orh.nhs.uk

David Shlugman
Nuffield Department of Anaesthetics
John Radcliffe Hospital
Oxford OX3 9DU
United Kingdom
E-mail: david.shlugman@orh.nhs.uk

Liz Soilleux
Department of Cellular Pathology
John Radcliffe Hospital
Headington
Oxford OX3 9DU
United Kingdom
E-mail: elizabeth.soilleux@orh.nhs.uk

Denis Talbot
Cancer Research UK
Churchill Hospital
Oxford OX3 7LJ
United Kingdom
E-mail: denis.talbot@cancer.org.uk

Nick Willcox
Neuroscience Group
Weatherall Institute for Molecular Medicine
University of Oxford
John Radcliffe Hospital
Oxford OX3 9DU
United Kingdom
E-mail: nick.willcox@molecular-medicine.oxford.ac.uk

Synopsis

The critical role of the thymus within the immune system is becoming increasingly well understood. Much of this knowledge is widely dispersed within the journals. Although thymectomy is well established as a surgical procedure, these advances need to be made available to the surgeon in a readily digestible form. In contrast, neurologists and physicians require a better understanding of the surgical aspects of the thymus. This book aims to provide an up-to-date and concise review of the thymus gland by including chapters, written by selected experts, for both the surgeon and physician in a brief and attractive manner. Our intention was not to produce a reference textbook but to provide a comprehensive, readily accessible guide for those interested in the field, with a specific description of the Oxford surgical outlook of the thymus.

K. Anastasiadis
C. Ratnatunga

Kyriakos Anastasiadis and Chandi Ratnatunga

Ignored for many years, it is only recently that the main role of the thymus has been established. The fact that the gland degenerates progressively with time and that its location appears to isolate it from a functional role in human physiology has contributed to this ignorance.

In the first century A.D. Rufus from Ephesus was the first to mention the thymus as a gland. In the second century it was described by the Greek physician Galen as "the seat of courage". The name of the gland is probably derived from the Greek. Pronounced differently in Greek, it means anger, and is synonymous with the notion of spirit. The ancients believed the gland was the emotional centre of the body, and some philosophers even described it as the abode of the soul. Latin provides an alternate etymological derivation. The Latin word for the herb with flowers shaped like the gland is "thyme".

With time it became accepted that the thymus had no specific role. In the sixteenth century Ambroise Pare described it as an excrescence. In the Renaissance there were several attempts to identify its role; it was described as a cushion to prevent damage to the heart or over-expansion of the lungs in the newborn, as a key organ in blood formation in the foetus and as the control centre of the body's metabolism. During this period, the gland began to appear as an organ in anatomic atlases. The first pathological role of the gland was proposed in the seventeenth century, when the Swiss physician Felix Platter described a case of suffocation caused by the compression of the trachea by the thymus. Indeed, Rehn performed transcervical exothymopexy in 1896 on a patient suffering episodes of suffocation. Later, Oppenheim in 1889 and Weigert in 1901 described thymic tumours in autopsies. Thymectomy was initially reported by Sauerbruch (Fig. 1) in 1912. By 1936, Blalock (Fig. 2) had performed the first successful thymectomy for thymic tumour, ushering in the era of modern thymic surgery. He also suggested thymectomy in the treatment of non-thymomatous patients with myasthenia gravis.

By the late 1950s and early 1960s the role of the thymus as a lymphoid organ became clearer from observations

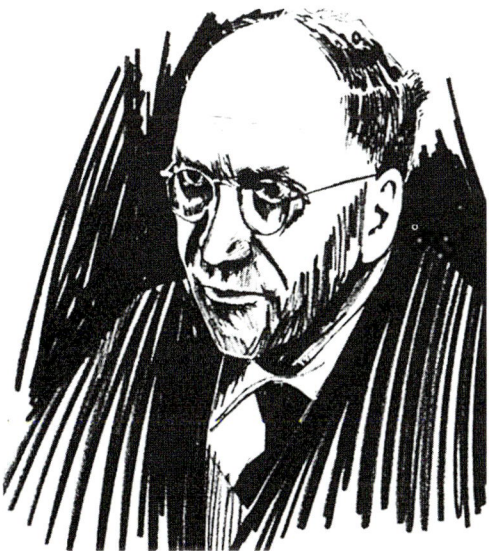

Fig. 1 Dr. Ernst Ferdinand Sauerbruch (1875–1951)

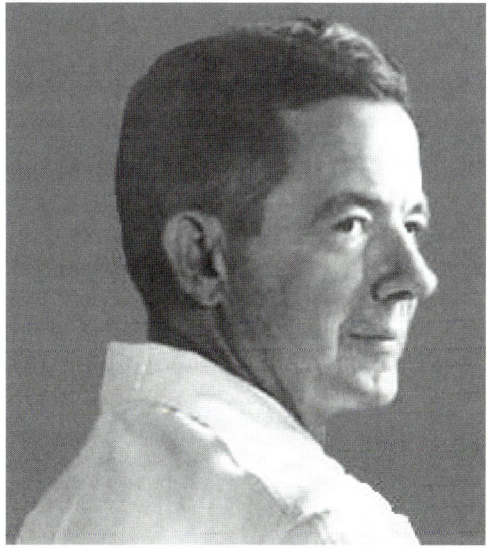

Fig. 2 Dr. Alfred Blalock (1899–1964)

of a decreased immune response and a consequently lowered resistance to disease that resulted from damage to or experimental removal of the gland. In 1954, Good described a patient with thymoma and immunodeficiency. In 1961, Miller showed that thymectomy in newborn mice resulted in immune-deficient animals, and this work sowed the seeds for our modern understanding of thymic physiology. Later, the hormone thymosin, derived from the thymus, was discovered and a possible endocrine role for the gland was also proposed.

In the 1970s, monoclonal antibodies allowed for the division of the immune system into humeral and thymic components, and the precise identification of the T cell subsets in the gland. Advances in research techniques, especially on a molecular basis, in myasthenia gravis and HIV contributed to a better understanding of the role the thymus gland and its physiology. The thymus became established as an organ with an integral role in the body's immune system. At the same time, thymectomy became increasingly performed for immunological rather than purely neoplastic reasons.

Our better understanding of thymic function led to the development of protocols for the management of patients undergoing thymectomy. This book sets out a surgical perspective to the thymus by providing a comprehensive up-to-date review of our scientific and clinical knowledge.

Suggested Reading

Blakeslee D. The thymus and immunologic reconstitution. JAMA, HIV/AIDS resource (www.ama-assn.org), 1999.

Blalock A, Mason MF, Morgan HG, et al. Myasthenia gravis and tumors of the thymic region. Ann Surg 1939;110:544–561.

Blalock A. Thymectomy in the treatment of myasthenia gravis. J Thorac Surg 1944;13:316.

Cooper MD, Peterson RDA, Good RA. Delineation of the thymic and bursal lymphoid systems in the chicken. Nature 1966;205:143.

Diamond J. Behavioral kinesiology: how to activate your thymus and increase your life energy. 1st Ed. Harper and Row, 1979, New York, pp 128–129.

Good RA. Agammaglobulinaemia; a provocative experiment of nature. Bull Univ Minn Hosp 1954;26:1–19.

Henry K. The thymus–what's new. Histopathology 1989; 14:537–548.

Hong R. The thymus. Finally getting some respect. Chest Surg Clin N Am 2001;11:295–310.

Izard J. Introduction to the thymus. Microsc Res Tech 1997;38:207–208.

Kirschner PA. The history of surgery of the thymus gland. Chest Surg Clin N Am 2000;10:153–165.

Leonidas JC. The thymus: from past misconception to present recognition. Pediatr Radiol 1998;28:275–282.

Miller JF. Discovering the origin of immunological competence. Annu Rev Immunol 1999;17:1–17.

Miller JF. Immunological function of the thymus. Lancet 1961;2:748–749.

Anatomy

Kyriakos Anastasiadis and Chandi Ratnatunga

1

Location

The thymus gland is located in the anterosuperior mediastinum. It usually extends from the thyroid gland to the level of the fourth costal cartilage. It lies posterior to the pretracheal fascia, the sternohyoid and sternothyroid muscles and the sternum (mostly behind the manubrium and the upper part of its body). It is located anteriorly to the innominate vein and is found between the parietal pleura and extrapleural fat and central to the phrenic nerves. It lies on the pericardium, with the ascending aorta and aortic arch behind it, while in the neck it lies over the trachea. Parallel to the gland on each side lie the phrenic nerves, which converge towards the gland at its middle segment (particularly important issue in thymectomy procedures). The gland consists classically of two lobes, even though other lobular structures may be present (Figs. 1.1, 1.2). The thyrothymic ligament connects the upper parts of its lobes to the thyroid gland. A variety

of extensions of the upper lobes, as well as relationships to the innominate vein, have been described (Figs. 1.3). Thus, rather than being located in its classical anterior position, one or both of the upper lobe thymus may even lie behind the innominate vein. Moreover, it has to be noted that besides the classical location of the gland, ectopic thymic tissue could be found in the mediastinal fat of the majority of patients. This is now accepted as the normal

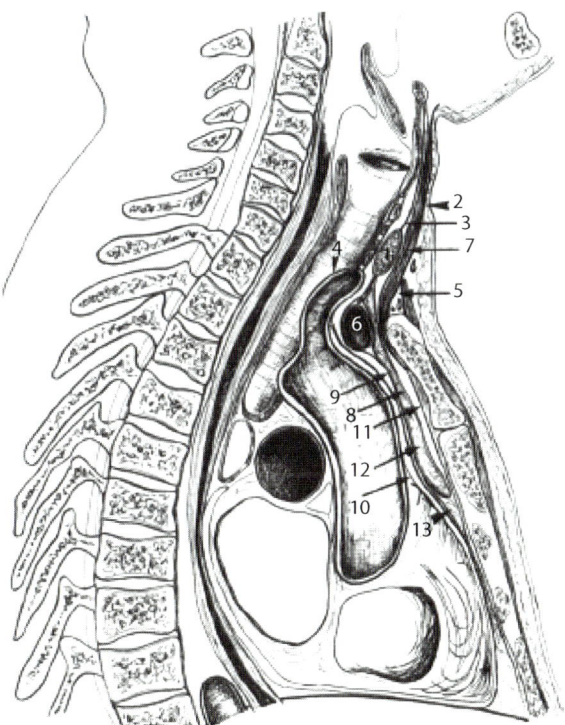

Fig. 1.2 Midline cervicothoracic sagittal section material demonstrating the thymus gland location (1=thyroid isthmus, 2=superficial layer of cervical fascia, 3=pretracheal cervical fascia, 4–brachiocephalic trunk, 5=pretracheal space, 6=left brachiocephalic vein, 7=sternothyroid muscle, 8=anterior wall of thymic sheath, 9=hyropericardial layer, 10=serous pericardium, 11=anterior interpleural ligament, 12=thymus, 13=subthymic fatty tissue) [1] (Used with permission)

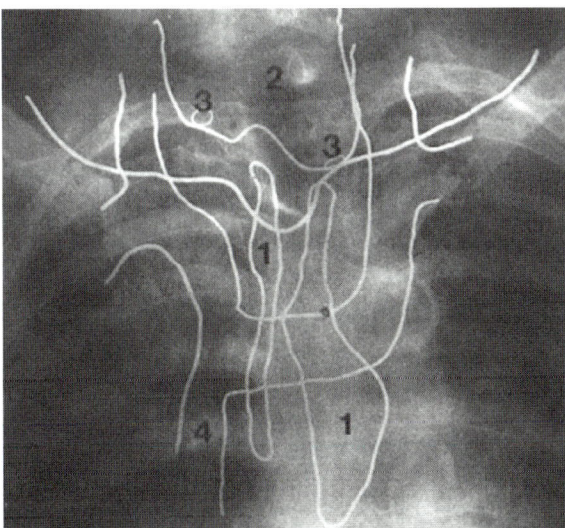

Fig. 1.1 Radiograph after outlining with radiopaque material demonstrating the thymus gland location (1=thymus, 2=thyroid gland, 3=parathyroid gland, 4=superior vena cava) [1] (Used with permission)

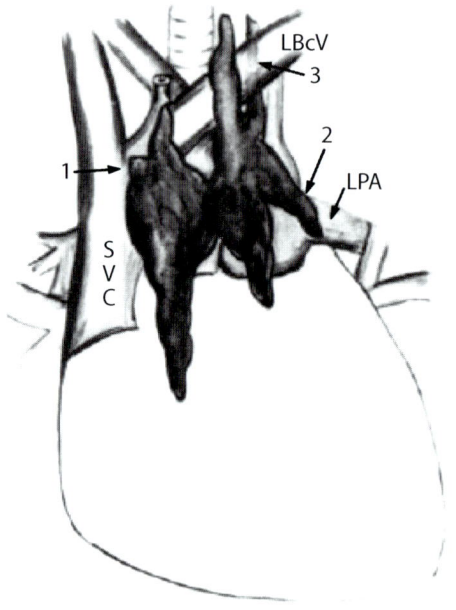

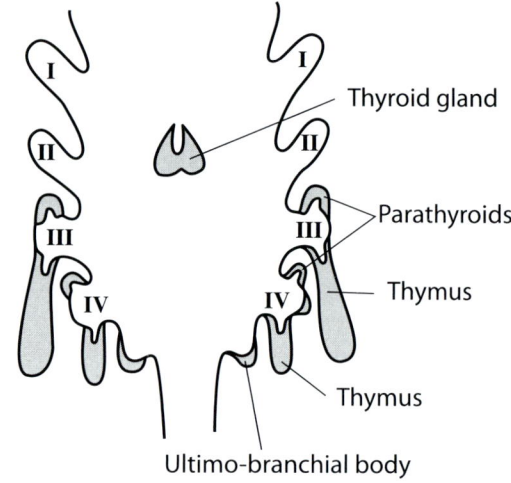

Fig. 1.4 Development of the brachial epithelial bodies [3] (Used with permission)

Fig. 1.3 Anterior and superior mediastinum show relations of normal thymus and variations to major vessels. *Arrows* 1, 2, and 3 show variable distribution of normal thymic tissue (LBcV, left brachiocephalic vein; LPA, left pulmonary artery; SVC, superior vena cava) [2] (Used with permission)

surgical anatomy of the thymus, defining the findings as "variation" and not "ectopic" [see chapter 9 – Fig 9.13, where a composite anatomy of the thymus as described by Jaretzki is illustrated, based on surgical-anatomical studies in 50 consecutive transcervical-transsternal maximal thymectomies for MG; thymic tissue was found outside the confines of the classical cervical-mediastinal lobes (A and B) in 32% of the specimens in the neck and in 98% of the specimens in the mediastinum].

Embryology

The thymus develops from the epithelium of the ventral diverticulum. It rises at the sixth gestational week from the third pharyngeal pouch and branchial cleft on each side as precursor to its ultimate bilobar structure, with possible minor contribution from the fourth pouch (Fig. 1.4). The thymic masses from each side move towards each other in the midline and come into direct contact, but do not fuse, remaining from the eighth week onwards as two connected thymic lobes. The gland then descends during the eighth week from the neck into anterior mediastinum of the thorax, to take up its final position.

The gland shares a common origin with the inferior parathyroids and the major thoracic vessels. Thus, parathyroid tissue can be embedded in the thymus, and a gen-

eral defect in the normal embryonic development of the thymus may involve anomalies of the parathyroids (i.e. DiGeorge anomaly) or major thoracic vessels or both. The stromal cell component of the gland that comprises of epithelial cells originates from the endoderm and becomes the thymic corpuscles (Hassal's) or the epithelial reticular cells. The connective tissue component of the gland is derived from surrounding mesoderm. The bone marrow donates the colonizing lymphocytes to it.

By the end of ninth week of development (see Chap. 3) the primordial thymus becomes competent to attract these lymphoid stem cells from the bloodstream, and to provide an epithelial microenvironment within which thymocytes can become mature T cells. The primary endodermal thymic cells are now infiltrated by lymphocytes of bone marrow origin, which undergo numerous mitotic divisions within the thymus and become the most numerous cell type in the organ. Appropriate development of the thymic epithelium during this period is important, as impaired development following neural crest ablation leads to loss of the gland's capacity to attract lymphoid stem cells.

During embryogenesis, failure of the gland to descend into the mediastinum or maldescent can lead to a partially (one lobe) or fully ectopic or to aberrant thymic tissue sequestration in the neck. This is not uncommon, and in only 2% of Jaretzki's and Wolff's patients was all thymic tissue confined to the thymic capsule. Ectopic thymic tissue in the mediastinum and in the neck has been described in up to 98% of the myasthenic population. This has important implications to thymectomy, as will be discussed in later chapters. Aberrant thymic tissue may, therefore, be found in the neck in up to one third of the population, as well as being dispersed in the mediastinum; common sites include lateral to the pleuropericardial surface in close proximity to the phrenic nerves, inferiorly adjacent to the diaphragm and the cardiophrenic fat, around the inferior pulmonary ligaments and also the pulmonary hilum or even the lungs. It can also be found in the sub-mandibular and paratracheal region, as well as in the aortopulmonary window or in the posterior mediastinum. Most of this ectopic cervical and mediastinal tissue, however, is cystic and non-functional.

Structural Anatomy

The thymus varies in weight and size with age. The adult gland generally weighs about 25 g and occupies an area of 25 cm³. It is pyramidal in early ages, but increasingly occupies an H-shaped structure in adulthood. It consists of two lobes, which are asymmetrical. It is pink-yellow, changing from pink in childhood due to its rich blood supply to yellow in adulthood due to adipose tissue deposition (Fig. 1.5).

The thymus is enclosed in a fibrous capsule that separates it from the surrounding tissues. Trabeculae originating from the capsule divide each lobe into multiple small structures, the lobules. Thus, thymus is a lobulated organ. These lobules are partially separated by a fibrous septum and are about 0.5–2.0 μm in diameter. They are composed of an outer layer, the cortex, which consists of epithelial cells of endodermal origin, and an inner layer, the medulla, which consists of epithelial cells of ectodermal origin and of lymphocytes. These epithelial cells form the framework of the gland, instead of mesenchyme, as is the case in other lymphoid organs. They are called epitheliocytes, and can be classified morphologically and functionally into six types. In the cortex they have a dendritic morphology forming a network that extends into the parenchyma of the gland. The space between them is occupied by lymphocytes.

The cortex is comprised of rapidly dividing, mainly small, lymphocytes called thymocytes, with a few macro-

phages amongst them. The medulla comprises medium-sized lymphocytes at a lower density, mature T cells and connective tissue. In the medulla there are also some other whorled structures of keratinised cells called thymic (Hassall's) corpuscles, which are composites of medullary epithelial cells and degenerating cell deposits. Their significance is still unclear, although recent data show that they participate in the physiological activities of the gland. The mature lymphocytes leave the thymus by entering the circulation from the capillaries within this layer and forming the circulating T cell population of the immune system.

Blood Supply

Arterial Supply

The thymus has no hilum and the arteries enter it through the cortico-medullary junction. It accepts branches from the inferior thyroid arteries, which rise from the thyrocervical trunk and from the pericardiophrenic branches of both internal mammary arteries, which rise from the subclavian arteries.

Venous Supply

The veins that accompany the inferior thyroid arteries and the pericardiophrenic branches of internal mammary arteries provide some venous drainage of the gland. The main venous supply, however, is central via veins in the posterior surface of the gland that run directly into the innominate vein. Alternatively, these tributaries form a common trunk, which flows into the innominate vein.

Lymphatic Drainage

There are no afferent vessels. Lymphatic vessels accompanying the arteries and veins drain the medulla and the cortico-medullary junction efferently into the mediastinal-brachiocephalic, tracheobroncial-hilar and internal mammary-parasternal nodes.

Nervous Supply

Sympathetic nerve fibres from the cervico-thoracic ganglion and the vagus nerve enter the gland following the route of the blood vessels. Phrenic nerve fibres are also distributed to the thymic capsule, forming neural plexuses at the cortico-medullary junction. The innervation of the gland is probably mainly for vasomotor purposes, but other roles, such as a neuroendocrine one, have been proposed.

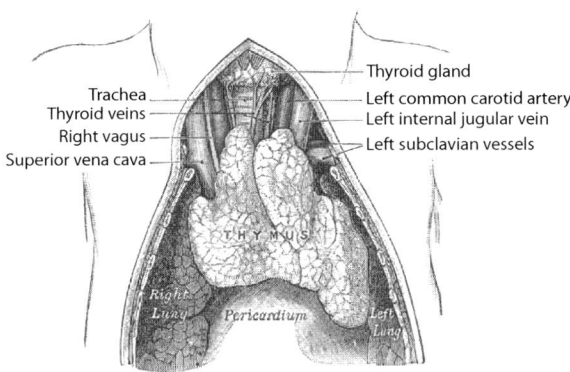

Fig. 1.5 The thymus gland during childhood [3] (Used with permission)

Suggested Bibliography

Banister LH. Haemolymphoid system. In Banister LH: Gray's anatomy. 38th edn. New York: Churchill Livingston, 1995, pp 1423–1429.

Bockman DE. Development of the thymus. Micr Res Tech 1997;38:209–215.

Bodey B, Bodey B Jr, Siegel SE, Kaiser HE. Novel insights into the function of the thymic Hassall's bodies. In Vivo 2000;14:407–418.

Jaretzki A III, Wolff M. "Maximal" thymectomy for myasthenia gravis. Surgical anatomy and operative results. J Thorac Cardiovasc Surg 1988;96:711–776.

Jaretzki A III. Thymectomy for myasthenia gravis; analysis of controversies regarding technique and results. Neurology 1997;48(Suppl 5):S52–S63.

Lele SM, Lele MS, Anderson VM. The thymus in infancy and childhood. Embryonic, anatomic and pathologic considerations. Chest Surg Clin N Am 2001;11:233–253.

Lumley JSP, Craven JL, Aitken JT. Thorax. In Lumley JSP, Craven JL, Aitken JT: Essential anatomy. 5th edn. New York: Churchill Livingston, 1995, pp 77–78.

Marieb EN. The lymphatic system. In Marieb EN: Human anatomy and physiology. 4th Edn. California: The Benjamin/Cummings, 1998, pp 751–752.

Martini F. The lymphatic system and immunity. In Martini F: Fundamentals of anatomy and physiology. 5th edn. New Jersey: Prentice-Hall, 2001, pp 760–762.

Moore KL, Dalley A. Thorax. In Moore KL, Dalley A: Clinical oriented anatomy. 4th edn. Philadelphia: Lippincott, Williams and Wilkins, 1999, pp 142–143.

Schurman HJ, Kuper F, Kendall M. Thymic microenvironment at the light microscopic level. Micr Res Tech 1997;38:216–226.

Sinnatamby CS. The thorax – Pt 5: anterior mediastinum. In Sinnatamby CS: Last's anatomy. Regional and applied. 10th edn. London: Churchill-Livingstone, 1999, pp 189–190.

Suster S, Rosai J. Histology of the normal thymus. Am J Surg Pathol 1990;14:284–303.

Van Wynsberghe D, Noback CR, Carola R. The endocrine system. In Van Wynsberghe D, Noback CR, Carola R: Human anatomy and physiology. 3rd edn. Boston: McGraw-Hill, 1995, pp 571.

Von Gaudecker B. Functional histology of the human thymus. Anat Embyol (Berlin) 1991;183:1–15.

References

1. Di Marino V, Argeme M, Brunet C, Coopens R, Bonnoit J. Macroscopic study of the adult thymus. Surg Radiol Anat. 1987;9:51–62.

2. Sone S, Higashihara T, Morimoto S, et al. Normal anatomy of thymus and anterior mediastinum by pneumomediastinography. Am J Roentgenol. 1980;134:81–89.

3. Gray's Anatomy of the Human Body. 20th ed. Philadelphia: Lea & Febiger, 1918; New York: bartleby.com, 2000.

Changes with Aging

2

Kyriakos Anastasiadis and Chandi Ratnatunga

The thymus gland is fully developed at birth and weighs about 10 g. It increases in weight until the age of two, when it plateaus, only to start increasing in weight again between the ages of seven and twelve. At this age its weight has doubled and it has become narrower and longer [1] (Fig. 2.1).

From then onwards throughout adulthood, there is a progressive replacement of the majority of the perivascular spaces with adipose and fibrous tissue. This process commences around middle age, and by the age of 50 fat accounts for more than 80% of the total thymic volume [2]. As a result, the thymus changes from a pink-grey gland to a yellowish mass that is difficult to distinguish from the surrounding mediastinal fat, and whose margins can only be determined by its capsule. This loss of working glandular tissue is described as "involution" and results in only a minimum of cortical or medullary tissue remaining in the adult gland. Others, however, have suggested that involution begins as early as birth and proceeds at a rate of approximately of 3% per year until middle age, when it slows to a rate of 1% per year. At this rate the thymus is projected to disappear at the age of 120 years [3–5] (Fig. 2.2).

This involution usually does not result in a change in the overall size of the gland. It is a controlled process

regulated by a number of gonadal and thymic hormones, and can be accelerated by adrenal corticosteroids and sex hormones [6–8]. Cytokines are also known to contribute to this process [9]. Experimental evidence suggests that thymic involution is neither intrinsic nor irreversible, but probably the result of age-related disruption of neuroendocrine-thymic interactions [10]. Thus, this process can theoretically be reversed by the neuroendocrine replacement of GH, TSH, T3, T4 and LH-RH analogues [11].

Functional Changes

Given that the thymus gland is the main site of T cell development and regulation of the body's immune system throughout life, the age-related changes of the gland are quantitative not qualitative and the adult thymus retains its ability to contribute to T cell reconstitution [12–16]. There is, however, a shift with age towards an increase in the number of activated or memory T cells, and an accumulation of cells that fail to respond to stimuli as efficiently as T cells from younger individuals [17]. Despite the decrease in thymic output with aging, however, there is a constant level of peripheral T cells. This is partly because the complete naïve T cell repertoire,

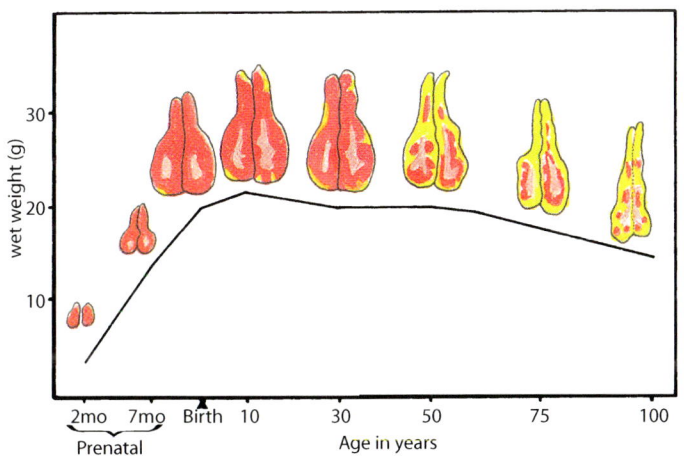

Fig. 2.1 The thymus changing with age [25] (Used with permission)

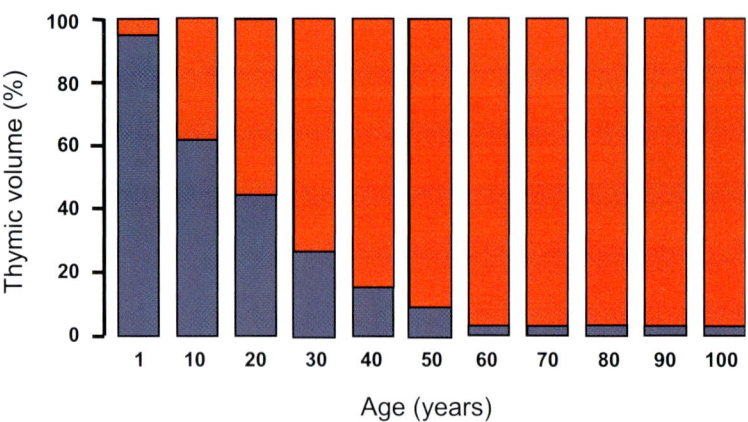

produced in the first year of life, survives throughout the life of the host and can, even in the absence of the thymus, maintain the body's T cell population [14]. T cell regeneration via relatively inefficient thymic-independent pathways [18] further complicate the constitution of this T cell pool. This aging process is gender-dependent. More recent thymic emigrants are found in older females than in older males [2].

Recent data, however, shows that the gland functions adequately, playing its role in optimising the immune system even into the sixth decade of life [19] and there are reports of the absence of complete thymic involution in thymic surgical samples of the elderly. The aging thymus retains the ability to stimulate naïve T cell recovery after bone marrow transplantation [20]. Adult thymopoiesis is also responsible for naïve T cell recovery in HIV-infected adult patients receiving highly active antiretroviral chemotherapy [21], and is essential for recovery of T cells after intense chemotherapy [14]. An increasing proportion of repletion of the T cell stock in aged patients, however, is also due to peripheral T cell expansion [12, 22].

The thymus, as described in the previous chapter, is influenced by the whole neuroendocrine system of the body, including the pituitary-thymic axis. The relationship between the pituitary and the thymus changes with age. Thymic development and aging is probably influenced by growth hormone from the pituitary gland, which is controlled by the hypothalamus. The initially positive signals from the hypothalamus just after birth decrease with age and are reversed around puberty, leading to the onset of thymic atrophy [23].

This impaired thymic function with advancing age may contribute to the increased morbidity and mortality in the elderly from infectious diseases, and possibly from autoimmunity and neoplasia [24].

References

1. Banister LH. Haemolymphoid system. In Gray's Anatomy. 38th edn. New York: Churchill Livingston, 1995, pp 1423–1429.
2. Steinmann GG. Changes in the human thymus during aging. Curr Topics Pathol 1986;75:43–88.
3. Pido_lopez J, Imami N, Aspinall R. Both age and gender affect thymic output: more recent thymic emigrants in females than males as they age. Clin Exp Immunol 2001;125:409–413.
4. Steinmann GG, Klaus B, Muller-Hermelinelink HK. The involution of the ageing human thymic epithelium is independent of puberty. A morphometric study. Scand J Immunol 1985;22:563–575.
5. Kendall MD, Johnson HRM, Singh J. The weight of the thymus gland at necropsy. J Anat 1980;131:485–499.
6. George AJT, Ritter MA. Thymic involution with ageing: obsolescence or good housekeeping? Immunol Today 1996;17:267–272.
7. Tolosa E, Ashwell JD. Neuroimmunomodulation 1999;6:90–96.
8. Kincade PW, Medina KL, Smithson G. Sex hormones as negative regulators of lymphopoiesis. Immunol Rev 1994;137:119–134.
9. Haynes BF, Hale LP. The human thymus. A chimeric organ comprised of central and peripheral lymphoid components. Immunol Res 1998;18:61–78.
10. Fabris N. Biomarkers of aging in the neuroendocrine-immune domain. Time for a new theory of aging? Ann NY Acad Sci 1992;663:335–348.
11. Moll UM. Functional histology of the neuroendocrine thymus. Micr Res Tech 1997;38:300–310.
12. Douek DC, McFarland RD, Keiser PH, et al. Changes in thymic function with age and during the treatment of HIV infection. Nature 1998;396:690–695
13. Flores KG, Li J, Sempowski GD, Haynes BF, Hale LP. Analysis of the human thymic perivascular space during aging. J Clin Invest 1999;104:1031–1039.

14. Douek DC, Koup RA. Evidence for thymic function in the elderly. Vaccine 2000;18:1638–1641.

15. Sen J. Signal transduction in thymus development. Cell Mol Biol 2001;47:197–215.

16. Poulin JF, Viswanathan MN, Harris JM, et al. Direct evidence for thymic function in adult humans. J Exp Med 1999;190:479–486.

17. Aspinall R, Andrew D. Thymic involution in aging. J Clin Immunol 2000;20:250–256.

18. Mackall GL, Gress RE. Thymic aging and T-cell regeneration. Immunol Rev 1997;160:91–102.

19. Haynes BF, Sempowski GD, Wells AF, Hale LP. The human thymus during aging. Immunol Res 2001;22:253–261.

20. Douek Dc, Vescio RA, Betts MR, et al. Assessment of thymic output in adults after haemopoietic stem-cell transplantation and prediction of T-cell reconstitution. Lancet 2000;355:1875–1881.

21. Haynes BF, Market ML, Sempowski GD, Patel DD, Hale LP. The role of the thymus in the immune reconstitution in aging, bone marrow transplantation, and HIV-1 infection. Annu Rev Immunol 2000;18:529–260.

22. Haynes BF, Hale LP, Weinhold KJ, Patel DD, Liao HX, Bressler PB, et al. Analysis of the adult thymus in reconstitution of T lymphocytes in HIV-1 infection. J Clin Invest 1999;103:921.

23. Hirokawa K, Utsuyama M, Kobayashi S. Hypothalamic control of development and aging of the thymus. Mech Ageing Dev 1998;100:177–185.

24. Linton P, Thomas ML. T cell senescence. Front Biosci 2001;6:248–261.

25. Gray's Anatomy, 38th ed. New York: Churchill Livingston, 1995, picture 9.30, p.1430.

Physiology

Kyriakos Anastasiadis and Chandi Ratnatunga

3

Thymic physiology is complex and poorly understood. The thymus is the main site of T cell maturation and is also a ductless (endocrine) gland. It regulates the immune system from fetal life onwards. From the ninth gestational week, its epithelial primordium is invaded by pre-thymic precursor cells from haematopoietic centres (which later include the fetal liver and then the bone marrow) [1]. Under chemotactic stimuli, these progenitor T cells enter the gland through post-capillary venules, then migrate into the outer cortex before eventually maturing and moving into the medulla [2]. During this period they undergo mitotic division every 12 h and gradually develop into mature T cells, which enter the circulation through the post-capillary venules.

As they mature, the thymocytes rearrange the genes for their antigen-specific T cell receptors (TCR), which recognise peptide fragments of antigens bound by HLA-class I molecules (for cytotoxic (CD8$^+$) T cells) or class II (for helper (CD4$^+$) T cells). After the pre-T cell stage, immature thymocytes simultaneously display both CD4 and CD8 as well as CD3. Cells that can recognise self-HLA are "positively selected" by cortical epithelial cells; thymocytes with no specificity for self-HLA die by neglect (>80% of the total). Among the survivors, the helper subset loses CD8 and becomes "single CD4 positive"; in contrast, the cytotoxic T cells become single CD8$^+$. Thus, MHC class I is required for the peripheral accumulation of CD8 cells [3], while MHC class II affects the long-term lifespan of the CD4 cells [4]. These are CD4 and CD8 lymphocytes, which constitute the two major subsets of T lymphocytes. The CD3 chains associate closely with the TCR and help to transmit signals during the binding of the cognate peptide-HLA complex. This TCR binding process also occurs in all mature T cells. As they reach the medulla, any potentially autoaggressive T cells are deleted by apoptosis [5,6]; this "negative selection" is also called "central tolerance". From the arrival of the progenitors, the entire process takes about two weeks: the exported cells, which are the body's ultimate T cell repertoire, represent about 3% of the input CD4$^+$/CD8$^+$ thymocytes (Fig. 3.1).

When mature, the "naïve" T cells are exported at a rate proportional to the remaining thymic mass [7]. Export of these recent thymic emigrants (RTE) is probably maxi-

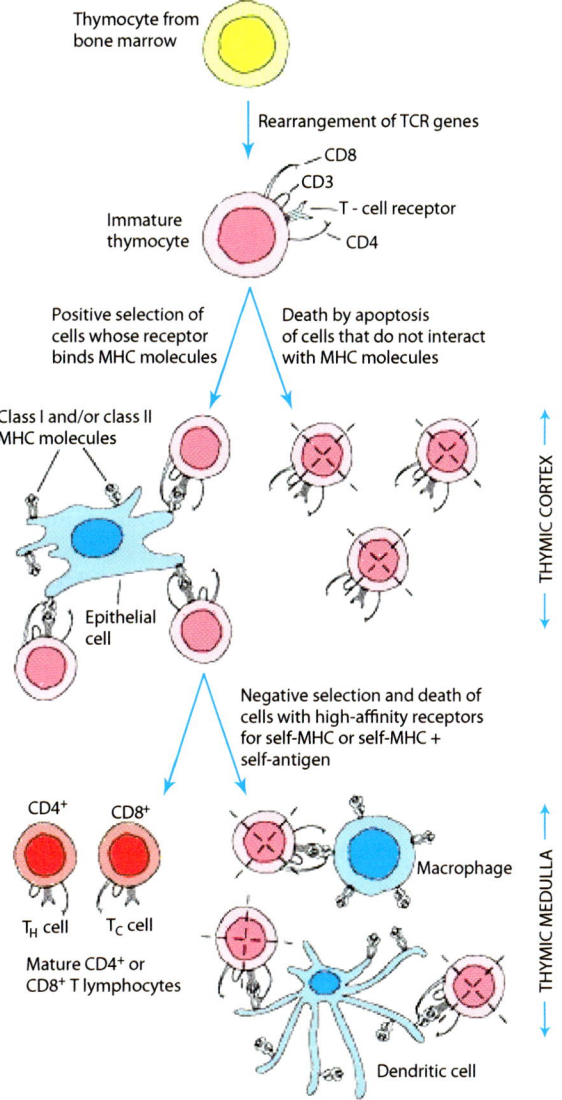

Fig. 3.1 Positive and negative selection of thymocytes in thymus (From *Kuby Immunology*, by Thomas J. Kindt, Richard A. Goldsby, Barbara A. Osborne. © 1992, 1994, 1999, 2003, 2007 by W. H. Freeman and Company. (Used with permission))

mal in early childhood, but continues at lower levels into adulthood and even middle age [6, 8, 9]. However, thymic output cannot be quantified in humans as there is no technique to differentiate RTE from long-lived naïve cells in the periphery. The increased thymic function during antiretroviral therapy for HIV infections, and after bone marrow transplantation and intensive chemotherapy, indicates that the adult thymus retains the ability to reactivate at least until age 40 or 50 (this may also be relevant to the growth of thymomas).

In the periphery, the RTE enter the lymph, blood and secondary lymphoid organs (spleen, lymph nodes, mucosa-associated tissue etc.), where they establish/maintain the peripheral T cell repertoire [2, 10–12]. After three to four weeks, those in surplus to what is required are discarded by unknown homeostatic mechanisms that can, on the other hand, allow small numbers of peripheral T cells to expand greatly if thymic output fails. Complete absence of the thymus (as in the DiGeorge anomaly), however, leads to a lack of thymus-derived T cell immunity [13–15]. Since there is very little, if any, extra-thymic generation of T cells [16, 17], cardiac surgeons should be less cavalier during preparation for cannulation for cardiopulmonary bypass when it is traditional in some quarters to remove thymic tissue and fat to gain access to the ascending aorta. An alternative strategy of retraction of this tissue, leaving the thymic tissue mass intact, is preferable.

In normal adults, CD4 and CD8 lymphocytes comprise around 60% and 30%, respectively, of the peripheral T cell pool, with a CD4:CD8 ratio of about 2.0 (ideally 1.74), which is similar to that among "single positive" thymocytes [5, 18]. In the periphery, the CD8$^+$ T cells depend on signals from HLA-class I to maintain a "foothold" [3], and the CD4$^+$ cells from class II to survive in the long term [4]. Many T cells have a prolonged wait before they encounter cognate antigen/co-receptor stimuli and proliferate [19]. During their subsequent responses they may release cytokines and/or mediate help (CD4 T cells) or cytotoxicity (CD8 T cells); afterwards, they either die or enter memory compartments [20].

Thus, this T cell antigen receptor (TCR) repertoire is established early in life. The increasing mass of the gland during the reconstitution of a lymphocyte depleted periphery may preserve the repertoire diversity and reduce the residual T cell clone expansion, while involution of the gland may reduce the homeostatic ability to maintain cell numbers in the elderly by T cell expansion [16]. A homeostatic mechanism maintains the peripheral lymphocyte pool size and is responsible for resident cell loss by random displacement or by selective loss of either RTE or naïve T cells or memory T cells, whenever an increase in the number of the peripheral pool occurs [21]. As mentioned above, this thymic output cannot be quantified in humans, as there is no technique to differentiate RTE from long-lived naïve cells in the periphery.

Although this output declines with the gradual involution of the gland, a substantial output is maintained throughout adulthood. With increasing age, however, this thymic contribution to the maintenance of the peripheral T cell pool declines and is replaced by peripheral T cell expansion [9].

The structure of the thymus ingeniously allows these essential subtle and complex interactions with the circulatory system to take place. Within the thymic cortex and medulla is the epithelial space, where thymocytes mature. The medulla contains another compartment called the perivascular space [2], which consists of connective tissue and which allows cells to enter or leave the medulla without passing through the cortex [22]. Lymphocytes (macrophages, plasma cells, eosinophils) are commonly found at this cortico-medullary junction of connective tissue. The basal lamina that separates these epithelial and perivascular spaces is called the "blood-thymus barrier", which prevents external macromolecules from entering the gland [23]. The thymus, therefore, never directly confronts circulating antigens, and thus avoids the activation of its immature T cells [1].

The adrenergic innervation of the gland has a modulatory function on immune cells and may play a role in the thymocyte traffic by controlling the thymic vascular tone. Catecholamines may also influence thymocyte development; so may neuropeptides such as VIP, tachykinins, calcitonin gene-related protein, enkephalin, somatostatin, chromogranin and synaptophysin. The pituitary hormones, adrenocorticotropic hormone (ACTH), thyroid stimulating hormone (TSH), follicular stimulating hormone (FSH), luteinizing hormone (LH), growth hormone (GH) and prolactin (PRL) are also thought to play a role in the gland's physiology, though this is not entirely clear [24, 25]. Data exist to show that GH stimulates intrathymic T cell traffic and, together with thyroid hormones, up-regulates thymulin production [26, 27].

Epithelial cells of the thymus gland secrete hormones that contribute to this process by stimulating the lymphocytes to become immunocompetent. These thymic hormones are: thymosin A, B1, B2, B3, B4 and B5; thymopoeitin I and II; thymic humoral hormone (THH); thymostimulin and thymulin or former factor thymic serum (FTS) [28–30]. They play a role mainly in the development of T cells into mature lymphocytes and some B cells into antibody-producing plasma cells [31]. Thymic epithelium and possibly even thymocytes, furthermore, produce steroids (glucocorticoids) that inhibit T cell activation and play a role in the control of T cell development [32, 33]; they may increase the TCR signalling thresholds required to promote positive and negative selection [34]. The relevance of these findings to humans, however, is not entirely clear.

Thymic development at the local level requires cellular interactions among thymic epithelial cells and thymocytes and other non-thymic mediators. Some of these have been defined as interleukins, colony stimulating factors, interferon gamma, thymosin alpha 1 and zinc thymulin [35]. Intracellular gene rearrangements and intercellular interactions during selection accompanied by cell proliferation, survival and death resulting in the maturation of thymocytes to T cells [36] is regulated both by thymic hormones and by cytokines (interleukins) [37, 38].

Thymic epithelial cells secrete many other peptides, which give them an endocrine and neuroendocrine role. Stimulated lymphocytes produce molecules similar to the peptide hormones ACTH, TSH, human chorionic gonadotrophin (HCG), endorphins and enkephalins [39, 40]. How these interact with non-thymic hormones and the precise role of non-thymic hormones in thymic function is far from clear. Somatostatin may play a role in thymic hormonal production [41]. Thymic endocrine function is up-regulated by thyroid and pituitary hormones, including thyroid hormone, PRL and GH [42, 43]. A hypothalamo-hypophyseal-thymic axis is present, which influences the production of thymic hormones and transmitters and, thus, regulates immune function [43–45]. A similar role may exist for the thymus-pineal axis [46]. Thymocytes produce vasoactive intestinal peptide (VIP), which is involved in thymic function [47]. There is also evidence that the thymus plays a role in somatic growth and differentiation, providing the stem cells for that [48]. Other non-immune roles have also been described: thymosin B4 and B5 influence hormones in the reproductive system.

Note: The authors are grateful to Professor Nick Wilcox for his helpful advice in constructing this chapter.

References

1. Von Gaudecker B. Functional histology of the human thymus. Anat Embryol (Berl) 1991;183:1–15.

2. Haynes BF, Hale LP. The human thymus. A chimeric organ comprised of central and peripheral lymphoid components. Immunol Res 1998;18:175–192.

3. Nesic D, Vukmanovic S. MHC class I is required for peripheral accumulation of the CD8 thymic emigrants. J Immunol 1998;160:3705.

4. Takeda S, Rodewald HR, Arakawa H, Bluethmann H, Shimizu T. MHC class II molecules are not required for survival of newly generated CD4 cells, but affect their long-term life span. Immunity 1996;5:217.

5. Sprent J, Kishimoto H. The thymus and central tolerance. Philos Trans R Soc Lond B Biol Sci 2001;356:609–616.

6. Res P, Spits H. Developmental stages in the human thymus. Sem Immunol 1999;11:39–46.

7. Gabor MJ, Scollay R, Godfrey DI. Thymic T cell export is not influenced by the periheral T cell pool. Eur J Immunol 1997;27:2986.

8. Berzins SP, Godfrey DI, Miller JFAP, Boyd RL. A central role for thymic emigrants in peripheral T cell homeostasis. Immunol 1999;96:9787–9791.

9. Haynes BF, Markert ML, Sempowski GD, Patel DD, Hale LP. The role of the thymus in immune reconstitution in aging, bone marrow transplantation, and HIV-1 infection. Annu Rev Immunol 2000;18:529–560.

10. Blakeslee D. The thymus and immunologic reconstitution. JAMA, HIV/AIDS resource (www.ama-assn.org), 1999.

11. Ropke C. Thymic epithelial cell culture. Micr Res Tech 1997;38:276–286.

12. Anderson G, Harman BC, Hare KJ, Jenkinson EJ. Microenvironmental regulation of T cell development in the thymus. Semin Immunol 2000;12:47–464.

13. Haynes BF, Sempowski GD, Wells AF, Hale LP. The human thymus during aging. Immunol Res 2001;22:253–261.

14. Withers-Ward ES, Amado RG, Koka PS, et al. Transient renewal of thymopoiesis in HIV-infected human thymic implants following antiviral therapy. Nat Med 1997;3:1102–1109.

15. Douek, Koup RA. Evidence for thymic function in the elderly. Vaccine 2000;18:1638–1641.

16. Sen J. Signal transduction in thymus development. Cell Mol Biol 2001;47:197–215.

17. Leclercq G, Plum J. Thymic and extrathymic T cell development. Leukemia 1996;10:1853–1859.

18. Jimenez E, Vicente A, Sacedon R, et al. Distinct mechanisms contribute to generate and change the CD4:CD8 cell ratio during thymus development: a role for the Notch ligand, Jagged 1. J Immunol 2001;166:5898–5908.

19. Shen X, Konig R. Post-thymic selection of peripheral CD4+ t-lymphocytes on class II major histocompatibility antigen-bearing cells. Cell Mol Biol 2001;47:87–96.

20. Rodewald HR. Immunology: the thymus in the age of retirement. Nature 1998;396:630–631.

21. Berzins SP, Boyd RL, Miller JFAP. The role of thymus and recent thymic migrants in the maintenance of the adult peripheral lymphocyte pool. J Exp Med 1998;187:1839–1848.

22. Kendall MD. The morphology of perivascular spaces in the thymus. Thymus 1989;13:157–164.

23. Kato S. Thymic microvascular system. Micr Res Tech 1997;38:287–299.

24. Moll UM. Functional histology of the neuroendocrine thymus. Micr Res Tech 1997;38:300–310.

25. Hadden JW. Thymic endocrinology. Int J Immunopharmacol 1992;14:345–352.

26. Savino W, Smaniotto, De Mello-Coelho, Dardenne M. Is there a role for growth hormone upon intrathymic T cell migration? Ann NY Acad Sci 2000;917:748–754.

27. Savino W, Villa-Verde DM, Alves LA, Dardenne M. Neuroendocrine control of the thymus. Ann NY Sci 1998;840:470–479.

28. Van Wynsberghe D, Noback CR, Carola R. The endocrine system. In Human Anatomy and Physiology. 3rd edn. McGraw-Hill, 1995, Boston, pp 572.

29. Bach JF, Dardenne M. Thymulin, a zinc-dependent hormone. Med Oncol Tumor Pharmacother 1989;6:25–29.

30. Hadden JW, Malec PH, Coto J, Hadden EM. Thymic involution in aging. Prospects for correction. Ann NY Acad Sci 1992;673:231–239.

31. Batanero E, De Leeuw FE, Jansen GH, Van Wichen DF, Huber J, Schuurman HJ. The neural and neuro-endocrine component of the human thymus. II. Hormone immuno-reactivity. Brain Behav Immunol 1992;6:249–264.

32. Van Laethem F, Baus E, Smyth LA, et al. Glucocorticoids attenuate cell receptor signalling. J Exp Med 2001;193:803–814.

33. Tolosa E, Ashwell JD. Thymus-derived glucocorticoids and the regulation of antigen specific T cell development. Neuroimmunomodulation 1999;6:90–96.

34. Ashell JD, Lu FW, Vacchio MS. Glucocorticoids in T cell development and function. Annu Rev Immonol 2000;18:309–345.

35. Hadden JW. Thymic endocrinology. Ann NY Acad Sci 1998;840:352–358.

36. Schuurman HJ, Kuper F, Kendall M. Thymic microenvironment at the light microscopic level. Micr Res Tech 1997;38:216–226.

37. Ritter MA, Boyd RL. Development in the thymus: it takes two to tango. Immunol Today 1993;14:462–468.

38. Dardenne M. Role of thymic peptides as transmitters between the neuroedocrine and immune systems. Ann Med 1999;31(Suppl):S34–S39.

39. Moll UM. Functional histology of the neuroendocrine thymus. Micr Res Tech 1997;38:300–310.

40. Smith EM, Blalock JE. A molecular basis for interactions between the immune and neuroendocrine systems. Int J Neurosci 1988;38:455–464.

41. Ferone D, van Hagen PM, Colao A, Annunziato L, Lamberts SW, Hofland LJ. Somatostatin receptors in the thymus. Ann Med 1999;31(Suppl):28–33.

42. Savino W, Villa-Verde DM, Alves LA, Dardenne M. Neuroendocrine control of the thymus. Ann NY Acad Sci 1998;840:470–479.

43. Dardenne M. Role of thymic peptides as transmitters between the neuroendocrine and immune systems. Ann Med 1999;31(Suppl):34–39.

44. Renoux G. The thymic factor system. Biomed Pharmacother 1983;37:433–440.

45. Geenen V, Robert F, Defresne MP, Boniver J, Legros JJ, Franchimont P. Neuroendocrinology of the thymus. Horm Res 1989;31:81–84.

46. Cardarelli NF. The role of a thymus-pineal axis in an immune mechanism of aging. J Theor Biol 1990;145:397–405.

47. Delgado M, Martinez C, Leceta J, Gomariz RP. Vasoactive intestinal peptide in thymus: synthesis, receptors and biological actions. Neuroimmunomodulation 1999;6:97–107.

48. Drummond R. An analysis of thymic function and the possible role of the thymus in stem cell production. Med Hypotheses 1995;44:292–294.

Thymic Diseases

4

Kyriakos Anastasiadis and Chandi Ratnatunga

There are many thymic diseases, which may be either congenital or acquired. The major diseases are described below, except from myasthenia gravis, which is discussed in greater detail separately.

Thymic Aplasia

Thymic aplasia is an uncommon developmental anomaly of the thymus gland, which occurs in early embryonic life due to an embryogenetic process involving the fourth branchial arch or the third branchial pouch [1]. This may be the result of a number of different factors, including those with chromosomal, mendelian, toxic or metabolic origins. Thymic aplasia is commonly associated with other congenital anomalies such as the absence of parathyroid glands and abnormalities of the heart, oesophagus and face. This group of congenital anomalies were once known as DiGeorge syndrome, first described in 1965 [4], and more recently known as DiGeorge anomaly (DGA).

This clinical condition includes arhinencephaly, cleft lip, cleft palate, uvula or diaphragmatic abnormalities, hydronephrosis, malrotation of the gut and imperforate anus [2]. Type B interrupted aortic arch and truncus arteriosus account for more than half of the cardiac lesions seen in DGA [3]. Today, DGA is redefined as a member of the monosomy 22q11 disorder and is known as CATCH 22 syndrome (cardiac defects, abnormal faces, thymic hypoplasia, cleft palate, and hypocalcaemia resulting from 22q11 deletions) [4]. In DGA there is usually thymic maldescent, with the thymus being absent from the mediastinum, rather than thymic aplasia, which accounts for less than 5% of DGA patients [5]. In these patients thymic aplasia leads to a deficiency of the immune system and to recurrent infections, which result in a limited life span. In 10% of DGA patients [6] the T cell deficiency is so severe that it endangers life.

Thymic Hyperplasia

Thymic hyperplasia can result in either thymic medullary hyperplasia or follicular lymphoid hyperplasia. It is found histologically in up to 50% of normal-sized thymuses [7].

It can be idiopathic or secondary. True thymic hyperplasia is a rare thymic condition with prevalence in children or young males, and is usually not associated with concomitant immune disease [8]. Secondary hyperplasia has been reported as a rebound effect from anticancer chemotherapy [9], from treatment with steroids [10] or during recovery from thermal burns [11]. Secondary thymic hyperplasia can also be an endocrine-related condition. It is associated with hyperthyroidism (Graves' disease), where thymic thyrotropin receptors may act as auto-antigens in the pathophysiology of Graves' disease [12]. Thymic hyperplasia can also present with other endocrine abnormalities, such as ectopic ACTH production [13], sarcoidosis and Beckwith-Wiedeman syndrome in association with visceromegaly [14, 15]. As will be discussed in subsequent chapters, thymic hyperplasia is related to myasthenia gravis [16], with up to 65% of myasthenic patients demonstrating thymic hyperplasia [17].

Thymic hyperplasia can also produce symptoms from compression of adjacent structures. Respiratory distress, caused by an enlarged and hyperplastic thymus [18], was described as early as the seventeenth century. Associated systemic manifestations due to lymphocytosis and red cell aplasia have also been described [19, 20]. Often, however, the patient is either asymptomatic or experiences only minimal accompanying symptoms [21].

Since thymic hyperplasia can mimic other diseases such as lymphofollicular hyperplasia, thymoma, lymphoma and germ cell tumour [22], a fine needle biopsy may be required for the diagnosis [23]. In the asymptomatic infant with a diffusely hyperplastic thymus a period of observation is warranted. Surgical resection is only recommended if the mass continues to enlarge or if the child becomes symptomatic [24]. In the adult with symptomatic, non-endocrine, benign masses, surgical excision relieves the mediastinal compression [25], and in massive hyperplasia early resection may be undertaken for differentiation from malignant masses [26]. In endocrine-related hyperplasia other therapeutic strategies may succeed. The increased size and density of the thymus gland that occurs in patients with Graves' disease is reduced after treatment with anti-thyroid drugs, which results in a concomitant decrease in thyrotropin receptor antibody levels [10].

Ectopic Thymus

Ectopic thymic tissue may be embedded along the line of thymic descent from the third pharyngeal pouches to the superior mediastinum. It may be found as a mass in the neck of children (aberrant cervical thymus) [27]. It results from either a complete or partial failure of the gland's descent, or from its sequestration and failure to involve along this pathway [28, 29]. The ectopic thymic tissue undergoes hyperplasia during the first decade of life, or after vaccination or infection [30]. This ectopic thymic tissue accounts for 10% of solid thymic masses in the neck [31], but is also known to degenerate into cysts [30]. Very rarely, the aberrant thymus is located in the subcutaneous tissue or within the dermis (dermal thymus) [32].

Its presentation in infants or in children is usually as an asymptomatic swelling of the neck, which can cause symptoms of compression of adjacent structures, such as the trachea (stridor, chocking spells, dyspnoea) or the oesophagus (dysphagia) [33]. Malignant transformation of this tissue has been described [34] and surgical excision of the mass is, therefore, recommended after diagnosis [33]. Operative outcomes are excellent, with no reported recurrences [35]. Confirmation of the presence of a mediastinal thymus should be made prior to surgery to avoid future immune deficiency [29].

Thymic Cysts

Cysts in the thymus gland can be congenital or acquired. Ectopic thymic cysts in the neck are well described [27, 36, 37] and result from a persistence of embryonal remnants [38] as discussed above [39]. Acquired cysts can develop from the parts of the gland or from tissues of other adjacent glands such as the parathyroids [40]. They have also been reported following lymphoma therapy [41], after radiotherapy to the chest in such diseases [42], after thoracotomy [43], and in as many as 40% of thymomas [44]. Multiple cysts are usually induced by an inflammatory process. They contain clear, turbid or haemorrhagic fluid, and often filtrate and destroy the gland, which may result in decreased thymic function [45]. Multilocular thymic cysts following HIV infection [46] and Epstein-Barr virus infection as a result of the gland's response to infection (thymitis) [47] have also been reported [48] and commonly leads to involution and immune deficiency in the subject [49].

About 10% of thymic tumours are benign cysts. These simple cysts should be differentiated from the commonly presenting cystic thymomas [50, 51]. The isolated benign cysts are usually of little clinical significance, and can be ignored unless they produce symptoms of compression. The majority of the patients with multilocular cysts are also asymptomatic, and the lesion is commonly discovered incidentally on routine chest radiography. Presentation with acute symptoms such as chest pain, dysphagia and dyspnoea may occur, and complete excision remains the treatment of choice [52]. Even in asymptomatic patients, however, multilocular cysts require thymectomy because of the difficulty in the pre-operative differentiation of malignant thymoma from benign cystic degradation or even thymic tuberculosis [53]. In some resected samples, coexisting epithelial thymic tumours are found [39]. Recurrences of the cysts several years after excision have been reported [45].

Histiocytosis

The thymus may be involved primarily or as part of a generalised process in Langerhan's cell histiocytosis (histiocytosis X) [54], especially in children and young adults. Here there is histiocytic mass formation and progressive cavitation in the thymus leading to immune deficiency. Histiocytes are macrophages, which are a normal component of the thymus [55] and which are necessary for lymphocyte differentiation. Langerhan's cells may be associated with Hassall's corpuscles in the normal thymus. Increased numbers of Langerhan's cells have been reported in the thymus of myasthenic patients [56]. This increase in the microphage population results in the destruction of thymic epithelium [54] and an enlarged dysplastic gland [57], which may either be smooth or nodular and may contain cysts and characteristic calcification [58]. Such glandular damage leads to a reduction in the peripheral blood lymphocyte subpopulation and a deficiency in the immune system [59]. Although the disease can be self-limiting, chemotherapy usually produces a regression of the changes [60]. Occasionally, however, even intensive treatment is unsuccessful [61].

Thymic Tumours

Thymic tumours can account for up to 47% of the masses found in the anterior mediastinum in adults [62]. Their classification is described in Chap. 7. In children and young adults, benign tumours are commonly teratomas [63] or thymolipomas [64], which account for 2–9% of all thymic neoplasms [65] and are more common in young adults. Some of them are exceptionally large. They usually are incidental findings, but may present, like cysts, with symptoms of compression of adjacent structures (trachea, oesophagus, major neck veins).

The purpose of surgical removal of these tumours is two-fold: diagnostic because of the high rate of malignancy in thymic tumours after the age of 18 months, and therapeutic when the tumours are symptomatic. Due to their generally benign and non-invasive behaviour, thymectomy is usually adequate [66], but adherence to adjacent structures may make the procedure extensive [67].

In children younger than 18 months a strategy of close follow-up is appropriate, perhaps with a trial of cortico-steroids, and surgery is reserved for mass enlargement or symptoms [68]. Malignant thymic tumours of childhood are mainly Hodgkin's and non-Hodgkin's lymphomas [69], together with germ cell tumours, teratocarcinomas, choriocarcinomas and sarcomas [70, 71]. Hodgkin's disease is the most frequent lymphoma in the young thymus, which can be involved either primarily or secondarily [72]. Common symptoms include weight loss, malaise, fever and night sweats [73]. The prognosis of the patient is dependent upon the stage of the disease, which also determines treatment. Treatment follows the conventional methods used in treating lymphoma [74].

The whole spectrum of these tumours in adulthood is described in Chap. 7, and includes germ cell tumours (seminoma and non-seminomatous tumours) [75], sympathetic ganglionic tumours (neuroblastoma and ganglioneuroblastoma) [76], haemangioma [77], thymic carcinoids, melanoma [78] and thymic carcinoma. Germ cell tumours of the anterior mediastinum account for 7% of all germ cell tumours [79] and are mostly malignant in adults [80]. Thymic carcinomas have more malignant potential and encompass a wide histological range, including squamous, adenosquamous, adenocarcinoma, mucoepidermoid, clear cell, basaloid, metaplastic, sarcomatoid, carcinosarcoma, lymphoepithelioma and neuroendocrine carcinoma [81–84]. Well-differentiated squamous, low-grade mucoepidermoid and basaloid thymic carcinoma are associated with the most favourable prognosis [88].

The clinical presentation of thymic tumours in adulthood is similar to their presentation in childhood. In the adult, rare metabolic conditions such as inappropriate secretion of antidiuretic hormone have also been linked with thymic neoplasms, particularly neuroblastomas [76]. Thymic carcinoid is a primary neuroendocrine tumour of the gland [85], which occurs mostly in middle-aged men and has a poor prognosis, often representing as a recurrence and metastasis after resection [86]. These tumours are associated with multiple endocrine neoplasia (MEN 1) [87] in as many as 25% of the cases [88]. They are also related to Cushing's syndrome and ectopic ACTH production [89].

Management of these tumours is surgery to obtain both a diagnosis and therapy. In the case of benign adult thymic tumours, complete resection is adequate. With the intermediate malignant carcinoid, complete resection is also the management strategy of choice, with radiotherapy and chemotherapy reserved for subsequent recurrences [90]. Reported survival in the literature is 27–33% at 5 years and about 7% at 10 years [91, 92]. With thymic carcinomas accurate staging and multimodality treatment, including surgery, is appropriate [88].

Thymoma

The most common malignant tumour of the thymus gland that is derived from thymic epithelial cells is thymoma [93, 94]. It accounts for 10–15% of all mediastinal masses and 50% of all anterior mediastinal masses. Thymomas appear mostly in the fifth and sixth decade of life. Their strong association with myasthenia gravis (MG) is well established, with up to 60% of patients with a thymoma having myasthenia gravis [95]. In contrast, thymoma is found in only about 10% of adult myasthenic patients [17]. Their presentation in 40% of patients is due to accompanying paraneoplastic syndromes [94, 96] (Table 4.1). The remainder of patients are asymptomatic or have local symptoms of compression of mediastinal structures, such as chest pain, dyspnoea and cough. Recurrent laryngeal nerve or phrenic nerve palsy and superior vena cava obstruction may also occur. Presentation with pericardial or pleural effusions is indicative of a poor prognosis.

As described in Chap. 7, thymomas are classified into five or six types, and exhibit benign to highly malignant behaviour [97, 98]. The incidence of well-encapsulated benign thymomas is 40–75%. Malignant thymomas in contrast display macroscopic or microscopic invasion of the capsule and adjacent mediastinal structures. Malignant thymomas, furthermore, can metastasise to lymph nodes, lungs and distant sites such as bone, liver and brain [96, 99, 100, 101]. Staging of these tumours, therefore, must combine radiological, surgical and pathologi-

Table 4.1 Accompanying paraneoplastic syndromes of thymomas

Thymoma – Associated Most Common Paraneoplastic Syndromes
Systemic Syndromes
- Cushing syndrome (Endocrine disorders)
- Pure red cell aplasia, Pancytopenia (Hematologic disorders)
- Alopecia, Pemphigus (Cutaneous disorders)
- Hypercalcemia
- Pemphigus
- Acquired hypogammaglobulinemia
- Systemic lupus erythematosus (Connective tissue diseases)
- Multiple endocrine neoplasia (MEN)
Neurologic Syndromes
- Myasthenia gravis
- Neuromyotonia
- Rippling muscle syndrome
- Gastrointestinal pseudo-obstruction
- Autonomic neuropathy
- Stiffman syndrome
- Cerebellar: CV2 syndrome
- Encephalopathy
- Collapsin response-mediator protein - 5

cal data. From the several staging schemes in the literature, the one proposed by Masaoka et al in 1981 is the most efficient and simple [101]. The WHO classification reported previously describes types A, AB, B1–3 and C thymomas. Type A and AB thymomas (medullary and mixed thymomas) are clinically benign, type B1–3 thymomas (predominantly cortical and cortical thymomas and well-differentiated thymic carcinomas) show lower-grade malignancy and most type C thymomas (category II malignant thymomas) are highly malignant. Paraneoplastic MG occurs only in types A, AB and B1–3 thymomas [98]. The TNM staging of thymomas adds little further value and is not in current use (Table 4.2) [99]. For thymomas classification see also Chap. 7.

Current guidelines for treatment of thymoma include complete surgical resection and multimodality therapy with adjuvant radiotherapy or chemotherapy. Both might be used against advanced disease [102, 103]. The therapeutic strategy for thymomas is discussed in greater detail in Chaps. 9, 11 and 12. Following surgery for thymoma, extrathymic malignant lesions (mainly pulmonary, but also gastrointestinal, hepatic and breast, sarcomatous and haemopoetic) may develop later in up to 20% of patients [104, 105, 106]. Patients who have undergone thymectomy for malignant disease must, therefore, be followed-up closely for second primary tumour development [107, 108].

Table 4.2 The TNM staging of thymomas [99]

'TNM' Classification of Thymoma	
T factor	
T1	Macroscopically completely encapsulated and microscopically no capsular invasion
T2	Macroscopically adhesion or invasion into surrounding fatty tissue or mediastinal pleura, or microscopic invasion into capsule
T3	Invasion into neighboring organs, such as pericardium, great vessels, and lung
T4	Pleural or pericardial dissemination
N factor	
N0	No lymph node metastasis
N1	Metastasis to anterior mediastinal lymph nodes
N2	Metastasis to intrathoracic lymph nodes except anterior mediastinal lymph nodes
N3	Metastasis to extrathoracic lymph nodes
M factor	
M0	No hematogenous metastasis
M1	Hematogenous metastasis
Clinical staging	Stage I , T1N0M0
	Stage II, T2N0M0
	Stage III, T3N0M0
	Stage IVA, T4N0M0
	Stage IVB, any TN1M0, TN2M0, or TN3M0, according to the degree of lymphogenous metastasis, and any TxNM1 for hematogenous metastasis.

References

1. Thomas RA, Landing BH, Wells TR. Embryologic and other developmental considerations of thirty-eight possible variants of the DiGeorge anomaly. Am J Med Genet Suppl 1987;3:43–66.

2. Conley ME, Beckwith JB, Mancer JF, Tenckhoff L. The spectrum of the DiGeorge syndrome. J Pediatr 1979;94:883–890.

3. Hong R. The DiGeorge anomaly. Immunodefic Rev 1991;3:1–14.

4. Wilson DI, Burn J, Scambler P, Goodship J. DiGeorge syndrome: part of CATCH 22. J Med Genet 1993;30:852–856.

5. Hong R. The DiGeorge anomaly. Clin Rev Allergy Immunil 2001;20:43–60.

6. Hong R. The DiGeorge anomaly (CATCH 22, DiGeorge/velocardiofacial syndrome). Semin Hematol 1998;35:282–290.

7. Camera L, Brunetti A, Romano M, Larobina M, Marano I, Salvator M. Morphological imaging of thymic disorders. Ann Med 1999;31(Suppl 2):57–62.

8. Ricci C, Pescarmona, Rendina EA, Venuta F, Ruco LP, Baroni C. True thymic hyperplasia: a clinicopathological study. Ann Thorac Surg 1989;47:741–745.

9. Hara M, McAdams HP, Vredenburgh JJ, Herndon JE, Patz EF Jr. Thymic hyperplasia after high-dose chemotherapy and autologous stem cell transplantation: incidence and significance in patients with breast cancer. A, J Roentgenol 1999;173:1341–1344.

10. Pompeo E, Cristino B, Mauriello A, Mineo TC. Recurrent massive hyperplasia of the thymus. Scand Cardiovasc J 1999;33:306–308.

11. Gelfand DW, Goldman AS, Law EJ, MacMillan BG, Larson D, Abston S, et al. Thymic hyperplasia in children recovering from thermal burns. J Trauma 1972;12:813–817.

12. Murakami M, Hosoi Y, Negishi T, Kamiya Y, Miyashita K, Yamada M, et al. Thymic hyperplasia in patients with Graves' disease. Identification of thyrotropin receptors in human thymus. J Clin Invest 1996;98:2228–2234.

13. Ohta K, Shichiri M, Kameya T, Matsubara O, Imai T, Marumo F, et al. Thymic hyperplasia as a source of ectopic ACTH production. Endocr J 2000;47:487–492.

14. Balcom RJ, Hakanson DO, Werner A, Gordon LP. Massive thymic hyperplasia in an infant with Beckwith–Wiedmann syndrome. Arch Pathol Lab Med 1985;109:153–155.

15. Hofmann WJ, Moller P, Otto HF. Thymic hyperplasia. I. True thymic hyperplasia. Review of the literature. Klin Wochenschr 1987;65:49–52.

16. Roxanis I, Micklem K, Willcox N. True epithelial hyperplasia in the thymus of early-onset myasthenia gravis patients: implications for immunopathogenesis. J Neuroimmunol 2001;112:163–173.

17. Wilins EW, Edmunds LH, Castleman B. Cases of thymoma at the Massachusetts General Hospital. J Thorac Cardiovasc Surg 1966;52:322–330.

18. Dimitriou G, Greenough A, Rafferty G, Rennie J, Karani J. Respiratory distress in a neonate with an enlarged thymus. Eur J Ped 2000;159:237–238.

19. Katz SM, Chatten J, Bishop HC, Rosenblum H. Report of a case of gross thymic hyperplasia in a child. Am J Clin Pathol 1977;68:786–790.

20. Konstantopoulos K, Androulaki A, Aessopos A, Patsouris E, Dosios TH, Psychogios A, et al. Pure red cell aplasia associated with true thymic hyperplasia. Hum Pathol 1995;26:1160–1162.

21. Rice HE, Flake AW, Hori T, Galy A, Verhoogen RH. Massive thymic hyperplasia: characterization of a rare mediastinal mass. J Pediatr Surg 1994;29:1561–1564.

22. Hoerl HD, Wojtowycz M, Gallagher HA, Kurtycz DF. Cytologic diagnosis of the true thymic hyperplasia by combined radiologic imaging and aspiration cytology: a case report including flow cytometric analysis. Diagn Cytopathol 2000;23:417–421.

23. Bangerter M, Behnisch W, Griesshammer M. Mediastinal masses diagnosed as thymus hyperplasia by fine needle aspiration cytology. Acta Cytol 2000;44:743–747.

24. Midulla PS, Dolgin SE, Shlasko E. The thymus. Pediatric surgical aspects. Chest Surg Clin North Am 2001;11:255–267.

25. Linegar AG, Odell JA, Fennell WM, Close PM, De Groot MK, Casserly DR, et al. Massive thymic hyperplasia. Ann Thorac Surg 1993 May;55(5):1197–1201.

26. Pompeo E, Cristino B, Mauriello A, Mineo TC. Recurrent massive hyperplasia of the thymus. Scand Cardiovasc J 1999;33:306–308.

27. Ellis HA. Cervical thymic cyst. Br J Surg 1967;54:17–20.

28. Shah SS, Lai SY, Ruchelli E, Kazahaya K, Mahboubi S. Retropharyngeal aberrant thymus. Pediatrics 2001;108:94.

29. Lundeen BE, Sty JR. Ectopic cervical thymus: a rare neck mass in an infant. J Clin Ultrasound 1994;22:412–415.

30. Loney DA, Bauman NM. Ectopic cervical thymic masses in infants. A case report and review of literature. Int J pediatr Otorhinolaryngol 1998;43:77–84.

31. Barrik B, O'Kell RT. Thymic cysts and remnant cervical thymus. J Pediatr Surg 1969;4:355–357.

32. Hiraumi H, Tabuchi K, Kitajiri S. Dermal thymus: case report and review of literature. Am J Otolaryngol 2001;22:294–296.

33. Baek C, Ryu J, Yun J, Chu K. Abberant cervical thymus: a case report and review of literature. Int J Pediatr Otorhinolaryngol 1997;41:215–222.

34. Spigland N, Bensoussan AL, Blanchart H, et al. Aberrant cervical thymus in children: three cases report and review of literature. J Pediatr Surg 1990;25:1196–1199.

35. Kacker A, April M, Markentel CB, Breuer F. Ectopic thymus presenting as a solid submandibular neck mass in an infant: case report and review of literature. Int J Pediatr Otorhinolaryngol 1999;49:241–245.

36. Nguyen Q, deTar M, Wells W, Corbett D. Cervical thymic cyst: case reports and review of literature. Laryngoscope 1996;106:247–252.

37. Terzakis G, Louverdis D, Vlachou S, Anastasopoulos G, Dokianakis G, Tsikou-Papafragou A. Ectopic thymic cyst in the neck. J Laryngol Otol 2000;114:18–320.

38. Kondo K, Miyoshi T, Sakiyama S, Shimosato Y, Monden Y. Multilocular thymic cyst associated with Sjögren's Syndrome. Ann Thorac Surg 2001;72:1367–1369.

39. Nguyen Q, deTar M, Wells W, Crockett D. Cervical thymic cyst: case reports and review of the literature. Laryngoscope 1996;106:247–252.

40. McCluggage WG, Russell CF, Toner PG. Parathyroid cyst of the thymus. Thorax 1995;50:913–914.

41. Borna-Pignatti C, Andreis IB, Rugolotto S, Balter R, Bontempini L. Thymic cyst appearing after treatment of mediastinal non-Hodgkin lymphoma. Med Ped Oncol 1994;22:70–72.

42. Linfords KK, Meyer JE, Dedrick CG, Hassell LA, Harris NL. Thymic cysts in mediastinal Hodgkin disease. Radiology 1985;156:37–41.

43. Jaramillo D, Perez-Atayde A, Griscom NT. Apparent association between thymic cysts and prior thoracotomy. Radiology 1989;172:207–209.

44. Gray GF, Gutowski WT III. Thymoma. A clinicopathologic study of 54 cases. Am J Surg Pathol 1979;3:235.

45. Suster S, Rosai J. Multilocular thymic cyst: an acquired reactive process study of 18 cases. Am J Pathol 1991;15:388–398.

46. Chhieng DC, Demaria S, Yee HT, Yang GC. Multilocular thymic cyst with follicular lymphoid hyperplasia in a male infected with HIV. A case report with fine needle aspiration cytology. Acta Cytol 1999;43:1119–1123.

47. Mishalani SH, Lones MA, Said JW. Multilocular thymic cyst. A novel thymic lesion associated with human immunodeficiency virus infection. Arch Pathol Lab Med 1995;119:467–470.

48. Kontny HU, Sleasman JW, Kingma DW, Jaffe ES, Avila NA, Pizzo PA, et al. Multilocular thymic cysts in children with human immunodeficiency virus infection: clinical and pathologic aspects. J Pediatr 1997;131:264–270.

49. Leonidas JC. The thymus: from past misconception to present recognition. Pediatr Radiol 1998;28:275–282.

50. Trastek VF, Payne WS. Surgery of the thymus gland. In Shields TW: General thoracic surgery, 4th edn. Baltimore: Williams & Wilkins, 1994, pp 1124–1136.

51. Hara M, Suzuki H, Ohba S, Satake M, Ogino H, Itoh M, et al. A case of thymic cyst associated with thymoma and intracystic dissemination. Radiat Med 2000;18:311–313.

52. Davis JW, Florendo FT. Symptomatic mediastinal thymic cysts. Ann Thorac Surg 1988;46:693–694.

53. FitzGerald JM, Mayo JR, Miller RR, Jamieson WR, Baumgartner F. Tuberculosis of the thymus. Chest 1992;102:1604–1605.

54. Bove KE, Hurtubise P, Wong KY. Thymus in untreated systematic histiocytosis X. Paed Pathol 1985;4:99–115.

55. Kyewski BA. Seeding of thymic microenvironments defined by distinct thymocytes-stroma cell interactions is developmentally controlled. J Exp Med 1987;166:520–538.

56. Bramwell NH, Burns BF. Histiocytosis X of the thymus in association with myasthenia gravis. Am J Pathol 1986;86:224–227.

57. Newton WA Jr, Hamoudi AB, Shannon BT. Role of the thymus in histiocytosis-X. Hematol Oncol Clin North Am 1987;1:63–74.

58. Heller GD, Haller JO, Berdon WE, Sane S, Kleinman PK. Punctate thymic calcification in infants with untreated Langerhans' cell histiocytosis: report of four new cases. Pediatr Radiol 1999;29:813–815.

59. Leikin SL. Immunobiology of histiocytosis-X. Hematol Oncol Clin North Am 1987;1:49–61.

60. Junewick JJ, Fitzgerald NE. The thymus in Langerhans' cell histiocytosis. Ped Radiol 1999;29:904–907.

61. Arico M, Egeler RM. Clinical aspects of Langerhans cell histiocytosis. Hematol Oncol Clin North Am 1998;12:247–258.

62. Mullen B, Richardson JD. Primary anterior mediastinal tumors in children and adults. Ann Thorac Surg 1986;42:338–345.

63. Bergh NP, Gatzinsky P, Larsson S, Lundin P, Ridell B. Tumors of the thymus and thymic region: III. Clinicopathological studies on teratomas and tumors of Germ Cell type. Ann Thorac Surg 1978;25:107–111.

64. Moran CA, Rosado-de-Christenson M, Suster S. Thymolipoma: clinicopathologic review of 33 cases. Mod Pathol 1995;8:741–744.

65. Shirkhoda A, Chasen MH, Eftekhari F, Goldman AM, Decaro LF. MR imaging of mediastinal thymolipoma. J Comput Assist Tomogr 1987;11:364–365.

66. Kitano Y, Yokomori K, Ohkura M, Kataoka T, Narita M, Takemura T. Giant thymolipoma in a child. J Pediatr Surg 1993;28:1622–1625.

67. Nichols CR. Mediastinal germ cell tumours. Clinical features and biologic correlates. Chest 1991;99:472–479.

68. Sauter ER, Arensman RM, Falterman KW. Thymic enlargement in children. Am Surg 1991;57:21–23.

69. Azuma E, Nishihara H, Qi J, Nagai M, Hiratake S, Zhang XL, et al. Thymic B cell non-Hodgkin's lymphoma in a child. Am J Hematol 1998;57:48–50.

70. Weidner N. Germ-cell tumors of the mediastinum. Semin Diagn Pathol 1999;16:42–50.

71. Iyer R, Jaffe N, Ayala AG, Eftekhari F. Thymic sarcoma in childhood. Br J Radiol 1998;71:81–83.

72. Strollo DC, Rosado-de-Christenson ML. Tumors of the thymus. J Thorac Imaging 1999;14:152–171.

73. Keller RI, Castleman B. Hodgkin's disease of the thymus gland. Cancer 1974;33:1615–1623.

74. Harris NL, Jaffe ES, Stein H, Banks PM, Chan JK, Cleary ML, et al. A revised European-American classification of lymphoid neoplasms: a proposal from the International Lymphoma Study Group. Blood 1994;84:1361–1392.

75. Moran CA, Suster S. Mediastinal seminomas with prominent cystic changes. A clinicopathologic study of 10 cases. Am J Surg Pathol 1995;19:1047–1053.

76. Argani P, Erlandson RA, Rosai J: Thymic neuroblastoma in adults: report of three cases with special emphasis on its association with the syndrome of inappropriate secretion of antidiuretic hormone. Am J Clin Pathol 1997;108:537–543.

77. Niedzwiecki G, Wood BP. Thymic hemangioma. Am J Dis Child 1990;144:1149–1150.

78. Fushimi H, Kotoh K, Watanabe D, Tanio Y, Ogawa T, Miyoshi S. Malignant melanoma in the thymus. Am J Surg Pathol 2000;24:1305–1308.

79. Dehner LP. Gonadal and extragonadal germ cell neoplasms in childhood. Hum Pathol 1983;14:493–511.

80. Nichols Cr. Mediastinal germ cell tumors. Clinical features and biologic correlates. Chest 1991;99:472–479.

81. Yoneda S, Marx A, Heimann S, Shirakusa T, Kikuchi M, Muller-Hermelink HK. Low-grade metaplastic carcinoma of the thymus. Histopathology 1999;35:19–30.

82. Negron-Soto JM, Cascade PN. Squamous cell carcinoma of the thymus with paraneoplastic hypercalcemia. Clin Imaging 1995;19:122–124.

83. Ritter JH, Wick MR. Primary carcinomas of the thymus gland. Semin Diagn Pathol 1999;16:18–31.

84. Dimery IW, Lee JS, Blick M, Pearson G, Spitzer G, Hong WK. Association of the Epstein–Barr virus with lymphoepithelioma of the thymus. Cancer 1988;61:2475.

85. Montpreville VT, Macchicarini P, Dulmet E. Thymic neuroendocrine carcinoma (carcinoid): a clinicopathologic study of fourteen cases. J Thorac Cardiovasc Surg 1996;111:134–141.

86. Soga J, Yakuwa Y, Osaka M. Evaluation of 342 cases of mediastinal/thymic carcinoids collected from literature: a comparative study between typical carcinoids and atypical varieties. Ann Thorac Cardiovasc Surg 1999;5:285–292.

87. Sugiura H, Morikawa T, Itoh K, Ono K, Kondo S, Kondo S, et al. Thymic carcinoid in a patient with multiple endocrine neoplasia type: report of a case. Surg Today 2001;31:428–432.

88. Tech BT, Zedenius J, Kytola S, Skogseid B, Trotter J, Choplin H, et al. Thymic carcinoids in multiple endocrine neoplasia type 1. Ann Surg 1998;228:99–105.

89. Gartner LA, Voorhess ML. Adrenocorticotropic hormone-producing thymic carcinoid in a teenager. Cancer 1993;71:106–111.

90. Economopoulos GC, Lewis JW Jr, Lee MW, Silverman NA. Carcinoid tumors of the thymus. Ann Thorac Surg 1990;50:58–61.

91. Wick MR, Carney JA, Bernatz PE, Brown LR. Primary mediastinal carcinoid tumors. Am J Surg Pathol 1982;6:195–205.

92. Fukai I, Masaoka A, Fujii Y, et al. Thymic neuroendocrine tumor (thymic carcinoid): a clinicopathologic study in 15 patients. Ann Thorac Surg 1999;67:208–211.

93. Moore KH, McKenzie PR, Kennedy CW, McCaughan BC. Thymoma: trends over time. Ann Thorac Surg 2001;72:203–207.

94. Morgenthaler TI, Brown LR, Colby TV, Harper CM Jr, Coles DT. Thymoma. Mayo Clin Proc 1993;68:1110–1123.

95. Furman WL, Buckley PJ, Green AA, Stokes DC, Chien LT. Thymoma and myasthenia gravis in a 4-year-old child. Cancer 1985;56:2703–2706.

96. Rosenow EC 3rd, Hurley BT. Disorders of the thymus. A review. Arch Intern Med 1984;144:763–770.

97. Debono DJ, Loehrer PJ. Thymic neoplasms. Curr Opin Oncol 1996;8:112–119.

98. Muller-Hermelink HK, Marx A. Pathological aspects of malignant and benign thymic disorders. Ann Med 1999;31(Suppl):5–14.

99. Yamakawa Y, Masaoka A, Hasimoto T, et al. A tentative tumor-node-metastasis classification of thymoma. Cancer 1991;1991:68:1984–1987

100. Lewis JE, Wick MR, Scheithauer BW, Bernatz BE, Taylor WF. Thymoma: a clinicopathologic review. Cancer 1987;60:2727–2743.

101. Masaoka A, Monden Y, Nakahara K, Tanioka T. Follow up study of thymomas with special reference to their clinical stages. Cancer 1981;48:2485–2492.

102. Graeber GM, Tamim W. Current status of the diagnosis and treatment of thymoma. Semin Thorac Cardiovasc Surg 2000;12:268–277.

103. Thomas CR, Wright CD, Loehrer PJ. Thymoma: state of the art. J Clin Oncol 1999;17:2280–2289.

104. Morgenthaler TI, Brown LR, Colby TV, Harper CM Jr, Coles DT. Thymoma. Mayo Clin Proc 1993;68:1110–1123.

105. Masaoka A, Yamakawa Y, Niwa H, et al. Thymectomy and malignancy. Eur J Cardiothorac Surg 1994;8:251–253.

106. Monden Y, Uyama T, Kimura S, Taniki T. Extrathymic malignancy in patients with myasthenia gravis. Eur J Cancer 1991;27:745–747.

107. Port JL, Ginsberg RJ. Surgery for thymoma. Chest Surg Clin 2001;11:421–445.

108. Pan CC, Chen PC, Wang LS, Chi KH, Chiang H. Thymoma is associated with an increased risk of second malignancy. Cancer 2001;92:2406–2411.

Myasthenia Gravis

5

Camilla Buckley

Introduction

Myasthenia gravis (MG) is included in this text because it is commonly associated with thymic pathology, and thymic surgery remains an important component in the management of patients with MG. MG can be inherited or acquired, but the genetic forms are rare and not associated with thymic pathology, so will not be considered here. The clinical features, patho-physiology and management of acquired MG will be described, with particular reference to the importance of the thymus.

Myasthenia Gravis is a prototype autoimmune disease, and is one of the best understood antibody-mediated disorders, with both the antigen (the acetylcholine receptor, AChR)) and pathogenic antibody having been identified more than 30 years ago. The characteristics of the antibodies and the mechanisms by which they cause the symptoms and signs of MG have been thoroughly elucidated.

The association between thymic abnormalities and MG has been recognised for more than a century, with the earliest description probably being that of Lacquer, who described a patient with MG and a thymic tumour [1]. It was soon recognised that patients with MG could also have an enlarged or hyperplastic thymus, and in 1917 Bell suggested that 50% of patients with MG had an abnormal thymus [2]. Current estimates are that 10% of patients with MG have a thymic tumour (thymoma) and 30% have a hyperplastic thymus, while 10% of patients with thymomas have MG.

Epidemiology

MGs frequently quoted prevalence of 10 cases per 100,000 people is probably an underestimate, as recent work has suggested significant under-diagnosis of it, especially in the elderly [3]. MG affects all races, with a constant worldwide prevalence, although the proportion of patients with each clinical subtype varies depending on location. The disease can develop at any age, but there are two peaks: in the second and third decade with a female predominance of 3:1, and in the sixth and seventh decade with a male predominance of 2:1.

Clinical Subtypes

MG can involve any skeletal muscle (generalised MG) or can be restricted to the extraocular muscles (ocular MG). Antibodies to the AChR are detected in 85% of patients with generalised MG and 50% of patients with ocular MG. In the UK, different antibodies to a muscle specific kinase (MuSK) are detected in 9% of patients with generalised disease, and are not found in patients with ocular MG. Thus, 6% of patients with generalised disease have no detectable antibodies, although the clinical features and response to immunosuppressive therapy is identical in these patients to those with identifiable antibodies, making it likely that they have as-yet undiscovered antibodies.

Patients can be further divided by age at onset and thymic pathology, which is useful clinically since optimal treatment varies depending on the subgroup, probably as a consequence of differences in underlying pathophysiology (Table 5.1). Early-onset MG patients are less than 40 years old at onset of disease, have AChR antibodies (usually at high titre), hyperplastic thymi, and are often female (male:female = 1:3). Late onset MG patients are more commonly male (male:female = 2:1), have atrophic thymi, and usually have lower titres of AChR antibodies. Patients with thymoma almost always have AChR antibodies, and can be any age at presentation, although they are often in their fourth or fifth decade. Patients without AChR antibodies were previously termed "seronegative", but with the recent discovery of antibodies to a MuSK in up to 40% of patients [4], they are now subdivided into those with and without MuSK antibodies, although the exact clinical features of the two groups have not yet been fully elucidated.

Pathophysiology

Neuromuscular Transmission

Since MG is a disorder of neuromuscular transmission, it is necessary to briefly review the physiology of the neuromuscular junction (NMJ) in order to understand the pathophysiology of the disease (Fig. 5.1). The NMJ

Table 5.1 Subgroups of patients with generalised MG applicable to UK population

MG subgroup	Age at onset (years)	Sex ratio M:F	Thymus[1]	Predominant HLA association	AChR antibody levels	Response of MG to thymectomy
Early onset	<40	1:3	Hyperplasia	B8 DR3	High	75% improve to a varying extent
Late onset	>40	2:1	Atrophy	B7 DR2	Low	No consistent improvement
Thymoma-associated	Any age	1:1	Thymoma	No consistent association	Intermediate	No consistent improvement
MuSK-positive	Any age	1:3	Normal or atrophy	Not known	Absent	No consistent improvement
MuSK and AChR-negative	Any age	2:3	Mild hyperplasia in some	Not known	Absent	Possible improvement

[1]Histological findings at thymectomy in the majority of patients

is specialised for neuromuscular transmission, with clustering of acetylcholine receptors and numerous folds in the muscle membrane to increase its surface area. When an electrical signal reaches the nerve terminal it causes release of vesicles containing acetylcholine (ACh). The ACh diffuses across the synapse and binds to AChR, triggering secondary processes that lead to muscle contraction. Release of each packet of ACh generates a miniature endplate potential (MEPP), and the summation of several MEPPs generates the endplate potential. Under physiological circumstances there is a vast excess of ACh released, and thus an inbuilt high safety factor for neuromuscular transmission exists. Acetylcholinesterase in the synaptic cleft rapidly degrades ACh, ensuring the muscle

response to each nerve impulse is rapidly reversed, and allowing the muscle to relax and be responsive to subsequent stimulation.

AChR and MuSK Antibodies

The nicotinic AChR is a 250 kD transmembrane glycoprotein composed of five subunits that spans the muscle membrane. The two ACh binding sites are located extracellularly, and when both sites are occupied the ion channel formed by the central pore transiently opens to allow the flow of cations into the muscle cell. AChR antibodies are usually of the IgG subclasses, and all four IgG sub-

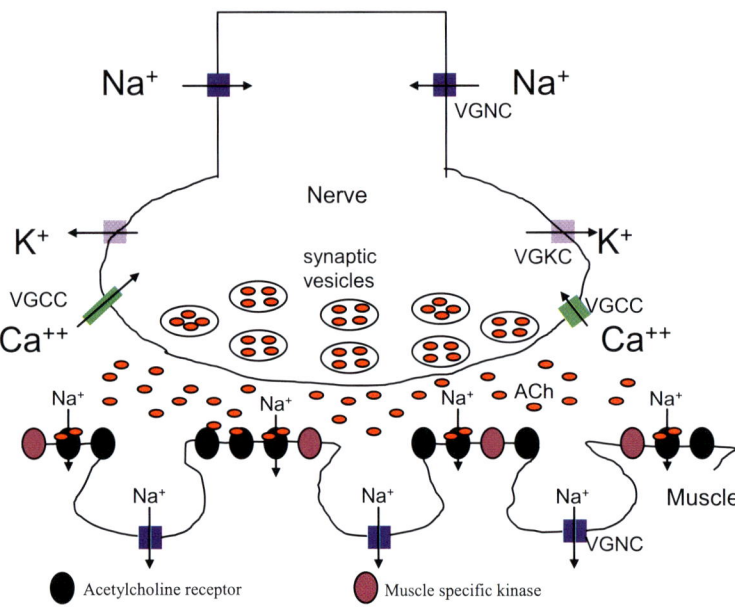

Fig. 5.1 Neuromuscular transmission (Ach, acetylcholine; VGNC, voltage-gated sodium channel; VGKC, voltage-gated potassium channel and VGCC, voltage-gated calcium channel)

types are represented, although IgG$_1$ and IgG$_4$ predominate. The antibodies have a very high avidity, with a K$_D$ of 5–100 pM, and are heterogeneous, binding to many different sites on the receptor. This heterogeneity may explain why there is a poor correlation between antibody titre and clinical severity across a population of patients with MG, but a relatively good correlation in the individual patient. Binding of the antibodies to AChRs dramatically decreases the efficiency of neuromuscular transmission by three main mechanisms: complement mediated damage to the NMJ; antibody-induced cross-linking of receptors accelerating endocytosis; and direct blocking of ACh binding.

MuSK is a receptor tyrosine kinase with four immunoglobulin-like domains, a cysteine rich extracellular domain and an intracellular kinase domain. It is expressed exclusively in muscle and is localised to the NMJ in mature skeletal muscle. MuSK antibodies are almost exclusively IgG$_4$ with some IgG$_2$. In vitro, they prevent agrin-induced clustering of AChRs, but their effect on adult neuromuscular transmission in vivo has not been fully elucidated.

The characteristics of AChR antibodies and the mechanisms by which they result in the clinical and electrophysiological features of MG are well defined but, as with the majority of autoimmune diseases, the processes that trigger the generation of these antibodies remain poorly understood. Identifying the factors involved is a priority, as it may lead to the development of more specific immunomodulatory therapies. The association between thymic abnormalities and MG, and the critical role the thymus plays in T cell maturation and development of self-tolerance, strongly suggest a role for the thymus in the generation of AChR autoantibodies. There is increasing experimental evidence supporting this hypothesis, and this evidence suggests that the exact mechanisms vary between the subgroups, as discussed below.

Patients with MG and Hyperplastic Thymus

Complimentary evidence from patients and animal models provides compelling evidence that the morphological changes in the hyperplastic thymus are relevant to the development of MG. T thymic cell cultures taken at thymectomy from patients with MG and thymic hyperplasia show spontaneous AChR antibody production in 65% of cases [5]. Moreover, the rate of antibody production in vitro correlates with serum titre of AChR antibodies and thymic histology [5,6], and the fine specificity of these antibodies closely match those found in the patients' serum [7]. The hyperplastic thymus is also enriched for AChR reactive T cells, and in patients thymectomised early there is a slow decline in the titre of antibodies following thymectomy [8].

In the animal model of MG, experimental autoimmune MG can be suppressed by total thymectomy [9]. If fragments of human hyperplastic thymus from a patient with MG are transplanted under the kidney of a mouse with severe combined immunodeficiency syndrome, then pathogenic antibodies to the human AChR are produced for several weeks after transplantation [10]. When MG is passively transferred to Lewis rats they do not develop germinal centres within the thymus, which implies that the thymic hyperplasia is not secondary to the autoimmune process, but is important in the initiation of the disease process [11].

Thymic myoid cells express the whole fetal AChR in its native conformation [12]. In the hyperplastic thymus the normal basal lamina between the germinal centres and the myoid cells breaks down, and there are numerous dendritic cells, macrophages and thymic epithelial cells that could act as antigen-presenting cells [13]. All the components required to generate an autoimmune response against the AChR are, therefore, present in close proximity. This leads to the hypothesis that in patients with hyperplastic thymus and MG, the thymus is the main site of production of autoantibodies to AChR.

Patients with Thymoma and MG

Thymomas are tumours of the epithelial component of the thymus that contain variable numbers of lymphocytes. They are unique among human neoplasms for their ability to generate mature T cells, and they have the highest frequency of associated paraneoplastic autoimmune diseases. MG is the most common of these autoimmune diseases, but haematological disorders such as red cell aplasia and hypogammaglobulinaemia also occur [14] (see Chap. 4). In the aberrant microenvironment of the thymoma there may be abnormal positive or negative selection, leading to the generation of autoreactive T cells [15]. Evidence supporting this comes from the detection of AChR epitopes in thymomas and the reduced levels of MHC 11 expression that are seen relative to normal thymic cortex [16]. Moreover, thymoma epithelial cells can express AChR peptides to T cell lines in culture [17].

Since the AChR molecule has not been detected in its native conformation, and B cells are rare in thymomas, it is assumed that these T cells migrate into the periphery, where they stimulate the production of AChR antibodies [18]. Evidence supporting this migration has been difficult to obtain, as the total peripheral T cell numbers are usually normal in patients with thymoma, and studies on T cell subsets have yielded conflicting results. Recent technological advances, however, have allowed the subset of peripheral T cells that have recently been exported from the thymus to be identified by the presence of T cell receptor excision circles (TRECs). Levels of TRECs are significantly higher in MG patients with thymoma than in all other MG patients, and these levels decline following removal of the thymoma but return to high levels if the thymoma recurs [19]. This provides strong support for the hypothesis that the thymoma exports unusually high numbers of T cells to the periphery, and it is assumed that among these will be potentially autoreactive cells.

The Role of Thymectomy in Management of Patients with MG

Patients with Hyperplastic Thymus and AChR Antibodies

This has been a controversial area ever since Sauerbruch, when performing a thyroidectomy on a patient with Graves' disease and MG, noticed that the thymus gland was enlarged and removed it, resulting in post-operative improvement in the patient's MG [20]. Although thymectomy has been part of the standard management of patients with MG since 1939, it has never been subjected to a randomised controlled trial. Furthermore, in the intervening years the medical treatment of MG has changed radically, with corticosteroids and other immunosuppressive agents becoming commonplace. Systemic corticosteroids dramatically alter the constituents of the hyperplastic thymus by markedly reducing the numbers of lymphocytes. A theoretical consequence of this is that there may be no additional benefit of thymectomy in patients already receiving immunosupression. This is very relevant to modern practice, as recent pilot studies have suggested that up to 70% of patients now receiving thymectomy are already on immunosuppressive medication.

The best assessment of the potential benefits of thymectomy in the modern era comes from a recent evidence-based review of 21 controlled but non-randomised studies published between 1953 and 1988 [21]. It demonstrated that patients undergoing thymectomy were twice as likely to attain medication-free remission, and 1.7 times more likely to show an improvement in their MG, but that there were too many confounding factors to generate a definitive set of guidelines for the role of thymectomy in the management of MG. The randomised, blinded, multi-centre international trial of thymectomy in MG being coordinated from Oxford aims to resolve some of these ongoing controversies. The trial is specifically designed to answer the question of whether there is still a role for thymectomy in the management of MG in the era of immunosupression (see Chap. 13).

Patients without AChR Antibodies

When thymectomy has been performed in patients without AChR antibodies, the thymus has usually been found to be atrophic, and there is no convincing evidence that there is any associated improvement in the MG symptoms. Some centres, however, still offer thymectomy to patients who do not have AChR antibodies. The picture has been complicated by the recent discovery of MuSK antibodies in some patients with MG but without AChR antibodies [22]. Pathological examination of the thymus in patients with MuSK antibodies reveals an atrophic thymus with no evidence of antibody synthesis within it. The histological appearance of the thymus in patients with MG without AChR or MuSK antibodies, however, demonstrates a milder version of the features seen in the hyperplastic thymus. The role of thymectomy in these patients, therefore, remains to be defined.

Patients with MG and Thymoma

There is no evidence that removing a thymoma has a beneficial effect on the prognosis of the associated MG in these patients. The indications for surgery, therefore, are purely for management of the tumour and are covered in other chapters.

Clinical Presentation

Patients with ocular MG have drooping of the eyelid (ptosis) and double vision (diplopia) (Fig. 5.2). In 60% of patients with generalised MG, these symptoms occur at presentation, but occur at some stage of the illness in 90% of patients, often accompanied by weakness of limbs, bulbar, or respiratory muscles. Fatigability is the classical feature of MG that helps differentiate it from other peripheral nerve and muscle disorders; hence, patients complain that they are weaker at the end of the day or after exertion. Symptoms are often worse following an infection, in hot weather or post-partum. There is an increased incidence of other autoimmune diseases, especially thyroid disease, in both the patients and their families.

Examination predominantly reveals proximal weakness with a predilection for facial, bulbar and neck muscles, with fatigability demonstrable on repetitive or prolonged testing of individual muscle groups. Weakness of respiratory muscles, especially the diaphragm, should be sought by observing for paradoxical breathing, and measuring vital capacity both lying and standing. The deep tendon reflexes are usually normal, as are sensory and general examination.

Diagnostic Tests

The diagnosis of MG is based on serology, electrophysiology and occasionally on clinical response to short-acting

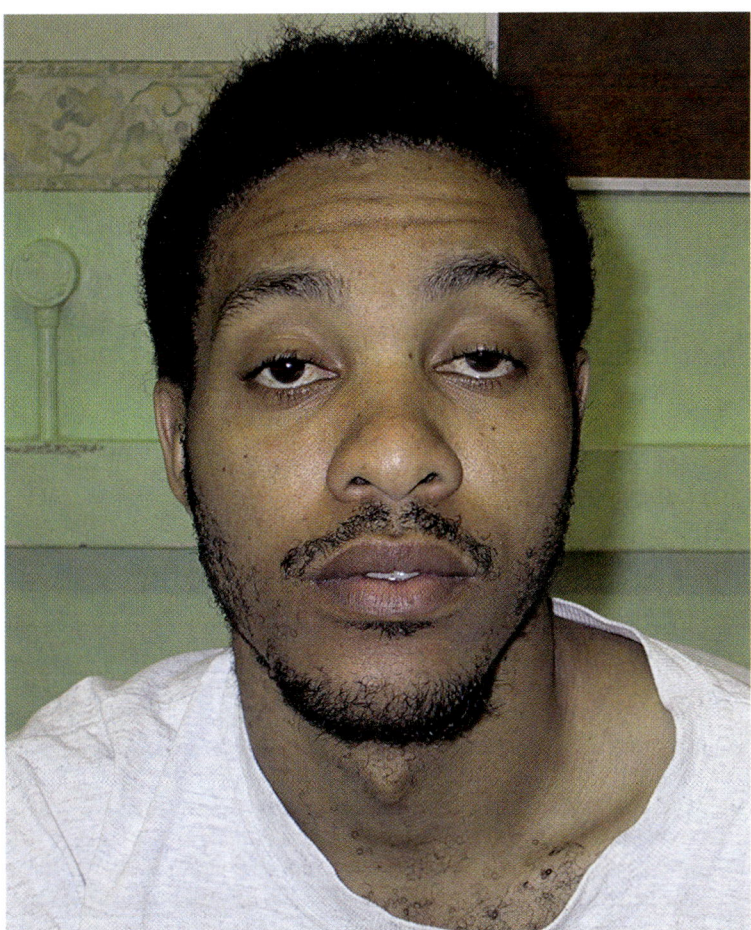

Fig. 5.2 Patient with newly diagnosed generalised myasthenia gravis at rest, demonstrating bilateral ptosis (drooping of the eyelids) worse on the left than the right, with overactivity of frontalis muscles in an attempt to compensate

acetylcholinesterase inhibitors. Antibodies to the acetylcholine receptor are detected by a radioimmunoassay with a specificity of >99%. The sensitivity is 85% for patients with generalised MG and 50% for patients with ocular MG. Antibodies to a muscle-specific kinase (MuSK) are detected either by radioimmunoassay or by ELISA in 9% of patients with generalised disease in the UK, and are not found in patients with ocular MG (22).

The classical electrophysiological feature of MG is increased decrement: on repetitive stimulation at 3 Hz there is rapid reduction (at least 15%) in the amplitude of the evoked muscle action potential (Fig. 5.3). A more sensitive test is increased jitter: when action potentials are recorded from pairs of muscle fibres innervated by branches of a single nerve fibre there is a time delay between the responses from the different muscles, a phenomenon known as jitter. The sensitivity and specificity of these tests is very dependent on the expertise of the neurophysiologist, but in experienced hands they approach that of serological tests.

In centres where expert electrophysiology or serology is not available, the "tensilon test" can be used. This involves objective documentation of a physical sign, e.g. ptosis, and assessing any change induced by an intravenous injection of edrophonium (a short-acting acetylcholinesterase inhibitor). In patients with MG there is a rapid and short-lived improvement in the physical sign. In Oxford, this test is rarely used due to the danger of precipitating a cholinergic crisis, even when the patient receives pre-treatment with atropine.

Treatment

A few patients with MG have symptoms that are so mild or intermittent that they only require symptomatic relief with acetylcholinesterase inhibitors. These drugs inhibit the activity of acetylcholinesterase, and thus prolong the time that ACh remains in the synaptic cleft at the neuromuscular junction before being metabolised. They can be given either orally or by subcutaneous injection, and patients usually notice symptomatic relief within 30 to 60 min of taking the medication. The effect persists for up to 4 h and so many patients take the medication five

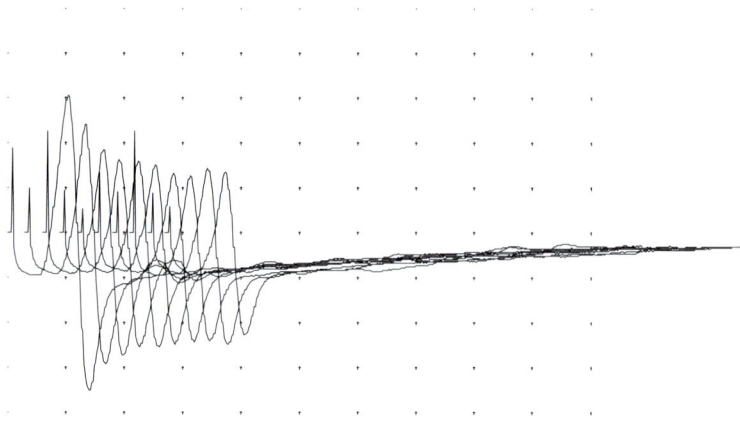

Fig. 5.3 Compound muscle action potential recorded during 3 Hz repetitive stimulation at supramaximal intensity, demonstrating decrement (reduction in the amplitude of the response with continued stimulation)

times a day. Theoretically, excessive doses of acetylcholinesterase inhibitors may be detrimental to neuromuscular transmission. The maximum dose recommended in Oxford is 60 mg five times a day.

The majority of patients will still be symptomatic on acetylcholinesterase inhibitor treatment alone and will usually commence immunosuppressant drugs. The first line immunosuppressive agent is the corticosteroid, prednisolone. Some patients deteriorate on starting prednisolone. To reduce this risk, the dose is usually titrated up slowly over two to three weeks to a dose of 1–1.5 mg/kg/day, taken on alternate days. If patients have significant bulbar or respiratory muscle involvement, they are admitted to the hospital for initiation of immunosupression to allow monitoring for deterioration and administration of acute therapy as required (see below).

The patient continues on 1–1.5 mg/kg/day on alternate days until they become symptom-free. The acetylcholinesterase inhibitor is then weaned and stopped. If the patient remains in remission the prednisolone dose can be slowly reduced (by 5 mg/month initially, and then by 1 mg/month when below 10 mg/day) to the minimum dose that maintains remission. Neurologists prefer to use an alternate day regime of steroids, as there is some evidence that this may reduce the incidence of side effects, especially of steroid-induced proximal myopathy. All patients need prophylaxis against corticosteroid-induced osteoporosis, and many will need proton pump inhibitors to protect them from the gastrointestinal side effects of steroids. All patients must be counselled regarding the common side effects of long-term corticosteroid use, namely osteoporosis, fluid retention and hypertension, increased appetite and weight gain, predisposition to infection, increased blood glucose, mood change, thinning of the skin, easy bruising and premature cataracts.

As the long term consequences of prolonged steroid use are being increasingly recognised, the majority of patients are increasingly treated with a "steroid-sparing agent" to reduce the cumulative steroid dose they receive. A randomised controlled trial performed in the 1990s clearly demonstrated that the cumulative steroid dose was lower in MG patients treated with prednisolone and azathioprine than in patients treated with prednisolone alone [23]. This effect was not apparent until patients had been taking azathioprine for more than a year. Although azathioprine is the first line agent, 10–15% of patients are intolerant of this drug, and in these patients cyclosporine, methotrexate and increasingly mycophenolate are used as alternatives. Thorough counselling of the patients and regular monitoring of blood pressure and appropriate routine blood tests are essential when using these "steroid-sparing agents".

Both plasma exchange and intravenous immunoglobulin (IVIg) are short-term treatments that are particularly useful in the management of a crisis or to optimise clinical function prior to thymectomy. Although both treatments are thought to be comparable, anecdotal reports suggest that some patients may respond to one better than the other. A typical course of plasma exchange takes five daily sessions and involves removing three litres of the patient's plasma each day through a femoral line and replacing it with 4.5% human albumin. Levels of antibodies can be rapidly reduced by plasma exchange, and improvement in clinical function can be seen within a few days and is maintained for six to eight weeks.

Several studies have shown temporary improvement in myasthenic symptoms, similar to plasma exchange, following administration of IVIg. The precise mechanism of action, however, remains unknown. A typical regime would be 0.4 g/kg/day of immunoglobulin administered by slow intravenous infusion for five consecutive days. Side effects of meningism, rash and hypertension are much less common with modern preparations, but since it is a blood product there is a theoretical risk of transmitting infectious agents.

Despite or in tandem with the above treatment strategies, thymectomy may be indicated for the patient (as discussed above). The preparation for surgery is critical in these patients to minimise the chances of perioperative myasthenic complications, and is further discussed in Chap. 10.

References

1. Laquer L. Beitrage zur lehre von der Erb'sche krankheit. I. Ueber die Erb'sche krankheit (myasthenia graics). Neurol Centralbl 1901;20:594–597.

2. Bell ET. Tumors of the thymus in myasthenia gravis. Jour Nerv Ment Dis 1917;45:130–143.

3. Vincent A, Clover L, Buckley C, Evans JG, Rothwell PM. Evidence of underdiagnosis of myasthenia gravis in older people. J Neurol Neurosurg Psychiatry 2003;74:1105–1108.

4. Hoch W, McConville J, Helms S, Newsom-Davis J, Melms A, Vincent A. Auto-antibodies to the receptor tyrosine kinase MuSK in patients with myasthenia gravis without acetylcholine receptor antibodies. Nat Med 2001;7:365–368.

5. Scadding G, Vincent A, Newsom-Davis J, Henry K. Acetylcholine antibody synthesis by thymic lymphocytes: correlation with thymic histology. Neurology 1981;31:935–943.

6. Newsom-Davis J, Willcox N, Schluep M, Harcourt G, Vincent A, Mossman S, et al. Immunological heterogeneity and cellular mechanisms in myasthenia gravis. Ann N Y Acad Sci 1987;505:12–26.

7. Heidenreich F, Vincent A, Willcox N, Newsom-Davis J. Anti-acetylcholine receptor antibody specificities in serum and in thymic cell culture supernatants from myasthenia gravis patients. Neurology 1988;38:1784–1788.

8. Vincent A, Whiting PJ, Schluep M, Heidenreich F, Lang B, Roberts A, et al. Antibody heterogeneity and specificity in myasthenia gravis. Ann N Y Acad Sci 1987;505:106–120.

9. Storb U. Steps in the generation of autoantibodies. Ann N Y Acad Sci 1993;681:29–32.

10. Schonbeck S, Padberg F, Hohlfeld R, Wekerle H. Transplantation of thymic autoimmune microenvironment to severe combined immunodeficiency mice. A new model of myasthenia gravis. J Clin Invest 1992;90:245–250.

11. Meinl E, Klinkert WE, Wekerle H. The thymus in myasthenia gravis. Changes typical for the human disease are absent in experimental autoimmune myasthenia gravis of the Lewis rat. Am J Pathol 1991;139:995–1008.

12. Schluep M, Willcox N, Vincent A, Dhoot GK, Newsom-Davis J. Acetylcholine receptors in human thymic cells in situ: an immunohistological study. Ann Neurol 1987;22:212–222.

13. Roxanis I, Micklem K, Willcox N. True epithelial hyperplasia in the thymus of early-onset myasthenia gravis patients: implications for immunopathogenesis. J Neuroimmunol 2001;112:163–173.

14. Souadjian JV, Enriquez P, Silverstein MN, Pepin JM. The spectrum of diseases associated with thymoma. Coincidence or syndrome? Arch Intern Med 1974;134:374–379.

15. Marx A, Schultz A, Wilisch A, Helmreich M, Nenninger R, Muller-Hermelink HK. Paraneoplastic autoimmunity in thymus tumors. Dev Immunol 1998;6:129–140.

16. Muller–Hermelink HK, Wilisch A, Schultz A, Marx A. Characterization of the human thymic microenvironment: lymphoepithelial interaction in normal thymus and thymoma. Arch Histol Cytol 1997;60:9–28.

17. Gilhus N, Willcox N, Harcourt G, Nagvejar N, Beeson D, Vincent A, et al. Antigen presentation by thymoma epithelial cells from myasthenia gravis patients to potentially pathogenic T cells. J Neuroimmunol 1995;56:65–76.

18. Vincent A, Willcox N. The role of T cells in the initiation of autoantibody responses in thymoma patients. Pathol Res Pract 1999;195:535–540.

19. Buckley C, Douek D, Newsom–Davis J, Vincent A, Willcox N. Mature, long-lived CD4+ and CD8+ T cells are generated by the thymoma in myasthenia gravis. Ann Neurol 2001;50:64–72.

20. Schumacher ED, Roth M. Thymektomie bei einem Fall von Morbus Basedowii mit Myasthenie. Mitt. Grenzgeb Med Chir 1912;25:746–765.

21. Gronseth GS, Barohn RJ. Practice parameter: thymectomy for autoimmune myasthenia gravis (an evidence-based review): report of the Quality Standards Subcommittee of the American Academy of Neurology. Neurology 2000;55:7–15.

22. Vincent A, Bowen J, Newsom-Davis J, McConville J. Seronegative generalised myasthenia gravis: clinical features, antibodies, and their targets. Lancet Neurol 2003;2:99–106.

23. Palace J, Newsom-Davis J, Lecky B. A randomized double-blind trial of prednisolone alone or with azathioprine in myasthenia gravis. Myasthenia Gravis Study Group. Neurology 1998;50:1778–1783.

Thymus and Thymoma in Myasthenia Gravis Patients

6

Nick Willcox

Introduction

The primary function of the normal thymus is to generate, select and export T lymphocytes – which it does during fetal life, childhood and even into the fourth decade [1, 2]. In general, T cell receptors (TcRs) bind antigenic peptide fragments presented by self HLA molecules; CD4+ "helper" T cells ([Th1]) are "restricted" to class II molecules (HLA-DR, -DQ or -DP), and CD8+ cytotoxic T cells to class I molecules (HLA-A, -B or -C). These highly polymorphic heterodimers differ most in amino acids lining their peptide-binding grooves, so the epitopes they present tend to show allele-specific binding motifs. In the thymic cortex, bone marrow-derived haemopoietic progenitors generate immature thymocytes in great numbers. As their TcRs rearrange, they generate a vast polyclonal repertoire with very diverse specificities for peptides/HLA variants. Those that can recognise peptides in the individual's own class I or class II alleles on the epithelial cells in the cortex are "positively selected" there, while the remaining 80–90% (that cannot do so) die by neglect [3].

The random process of TcR gene rearrangement inevitably generates some T cells with high affinities for self HLA molecules. So, as the surviving cells mature and move into the thymic medulla, they are "screened" for potential autoreactivity. When they encounter bone marrow-derived dendritic cells, macrophages or medullary epithelial cells at the cortico-medullary junction, those with autoaggressive potential are "negatively selected" (deleted). Occasional medullary epithelial cells express autoantigens from peripheral tissues, e.g. insulin [21]; they too may delete T cells with high affinities for their epitopes. As a result, the T cells eventually exported into the peripheral pool recognise self HLA molecules very weakly – except for those occupied by peptides (derived from foreign antigens) that have optimal contact sites for their particular TcRs. Finally, 5–10% of the nascent CD4+ T cells in the medulla develop locally into CD25+ regulatory T cells (T reg) that can dampen or suppress responses of other T cells and prevent them from expanding out of control [4].

"Myasthenia" means weakness of voluntary muscles, and results from defects in neuromuscular transmission. These usually cause loss of acetylcholine receptors (AChRs) on the post-synaptic (muscle) membrane; reserves of AChR are so limited in humans that a reduction of >60% is enough to cause weakness. In the rare inherited (congenital) myasthenias, there may be mutations in the AChR subunits or in adjacent proteins [5, 6]. By contrast, in myasthenia gravis (MG) receptor loss is caused by auto-antibodies specific either to the AChR itself (>80%), or (apparently) to the nearby muscle-specific kinase (MuSK) [7, 8]. These high affinity IgG antibodies can readily be detected in very sensitive and specific radio-immunoassays (RIAs), which are invaluable for diagnosis [9,10]; false positives are very rare. Currently, however, 5–10% of patients are negative in both assays. Since their typical generalised MG clearly improves on plasma exchange, they apparently have auto-antibodies to distinct neuromuscular target(s) whose identification is a high priority.

As reviewed in chapter 5, the weakness in MG is characteristically "fatiguable", meaning it increases with increasing effort. It usually first affects the extra-ocular muscles, causing ptosis and/or diplopia, which remain the only defects in ~15% of cases. In the other ~85%, the myasthenia generalises, usually within the next three years, to affect movements of the face, mouth, throat, neck and/or limbs [11]. More seriously, there may be problems with swallowing (even leading to inhalation pneumonia) and/or breathing (demanding assisted ventilation) so MG can still be life-threatening.

The AChR comprises two α subunits and plus single β, γ and δ subunits; the γ is replaced by an ε during the third trimester of fetal life. These subunits are all related in evolution [12]; each has about 210 extracellular amino acids, three transmembrane segments in close order, about 100 - residue cytoplasmic loops, a fourth transmembrane segment and a short extracellular C-terminal tail. Together, they form a channel with a central pore that opens when AChs occupy both of their binding sites at the α/δ and α/ε interfaces. The α subunit also includes major epitopes for MG auto-antibodies [13], though they are very hard to map because of the conformational complexity of the extracellular domain.

The anti-AChR antibodies in MG are almost entirely specific for extracellular epitopes in the native molecule [13]. They are mainly IgG1 and IgG3, and cause loss of

Table 6.1 MG Patient Subgroups

MG subgroup	MG[a] severity	M:F	Onset age	HLA	Auto- antibodies	Thymus
Ocular	I	3:2	2–80	none/clear	a-AChR⁺ or ⁻ (~55%) (~45%)	mild hyperplasia
Generalised anti-AChR seropositive						
EOMG	IIa-IV	1:3	10–40	**DR3, B8**	a-AChR⁺ (100%)	**hyperplasia**
LOMG	IIa-IV	3:2	> 40	DR2, B7	a-AChR⁺ (100%) titin, IFN-α, IL-12	normal/**atrophy**
Thymoma	IIa-IV	1:1	12–90	none clear	a-AChR⁺ (100%) **titin, IFN-α, IL-12**	**neoplasia +** adj. hyperplasia[b]
Generalised anti-AChR seronegative						
a-MuSK⁺	IIa-IV	1:3	2–65	?DR14	a-MuSK⁺ (100%)	normal/**atrophy**
a-MuSK⁻	IIa-III	1:2	10–70	not clear	target not clear	**mild hyperplasia**

features in **bold** are seen in the majority of patients in that subgroup

a-AChR, a-MuSK serum auto-antibody status

[a]MG grade: I, only extra-ocular muscle weakness; IIa, IIb and III, mild, moderate or severe generalised muscle weakness; the latter is acute in grade IV

[b]hyperplastic changes in the adjacent uninvolved thymus

receptors partly by accelerating their degradation, but mainly by activating complement; the ensuing damage tends to flatten the junctional folds in the muscle membrane and reduce total surface area [14]. Only a minority of antibodies in a minority of patients causes pharmacological blockage of ACh binding. The anti-MuSK antibodies are mainly IgG4, which does not activate complement, and their role in pathogenesis is not fully understood [10]. Nevertheless, they clearly identify a separate MG subgroup (Table 6.1) [15], and have not yet been detected in other patients with anti-AChR antibodies, with pure ocular MG, or with thymomas.

Classifying MG patients into subgroups is highly informative. Patients with early-onset MG (EOMG; onset before age 40) form a very distinctive subgroup in Caucasians. They have characteristic thymic changes, and are the likeliest to show benefits from thymectomy [16, 17]. Though these have still not been rigorously proven [18], many clinicians believe that the myasthenia remits in about a quarter of thymectomised patients (usually within 2–3 years), improves in about one half of patients, and is unaffected in the remaining quarter. The well known HLA-DR3-B8 associations are especially strong in the 70–80% of females [19]; since their EOMG almost always starts between puberty and menopause, hormonal influences seem highly likely. Autoimmunisation apparently involves the thymus, and may be a two-step process (see below).

The EOMG thymus consistently shows medullary lymph node-like infiltrates that expand from perivascular spaces and compress the epithelial cells into characteristic bands and cords [20]. Some of these epithelial cells express HLA-class II and sometimes also AChR subunits [21]; since they also bear CXCR13 and produce IL-6 [22], they may be well placed to attract and autoimmunise mature T cells (Step I) [20].

Rare nearby muscle-like thymic myoid cells are haphazardly scattered in the normal and EOMG medulla, and express striated muscle proteins; these include intact AChR of the fetal isoform that is often preferred by the patients' auto-antibodies [23]. The myoid cells are clearly implicated in provoking the infiltrates in EOMG, especially the germinal centres (Step II) [20]. Since these are the essential sites of all antibody mutation/diversification [24], it is no surprise that anti-AChR antibodies cloned from these thymi have proved to be highly mutated [25]; the very heterogeneity of the anti-AChR auto-antibodies may enhance their pathogenicity. There is also local activation of AChR-specific plasma cells, which are readily detectable in most EOMG thymi by their spontaneous production of anti-AChR antibodies, especially in patients with the highest serum anti-AChR titres [26].

If thymectomy does, indeed, prove to be beneficial, one might predict that its role is to interrupt the above steps in auto-immunisation.

Pre-treatment with corticosteroids can grossly deplete thymocytes, though the effects vary widely [27]. Since the cortex is especially steroid-susceptible, the medullary epithelium and the infiltrates often appear enriched, even though their total bulk is reduced [27]. Especially after steroids have been combined with azathioprine, the thymus may be so drastically collapsed as scarcely to warrant resection at all. Unfortunately, since it may then be replaced by fat, it is not possible to assess the completeness of this "hormonal thymectomy" radiologically, even with enhancement, so pre-operative measurement of residual thymus tissue is not yet possible.

In patients with neither anti-AChR nor anti-MuSK auto-antibodies, the thymus often shows changes very similar to those in EOMG; like their myasthenia, these are somewhat milder, with fewer, smaller, germinal centres, though similar infiltrating T cell areas are still obvious [28, 29]. Other hints that these patients belong to the EOMG spectrum imply that they too might benefit from thymectomy.

In most anti-MuSK⁺ patients, by contrast, the thymus appears normal for age or prematurely atrophic [28, 29], with little sign of past inflammation that has "burnt-out" later. The myasthenia is often predominantly bulbar, with respiratory crises in 30–40% [30]. It appears not to respond to thymectomy, and is often also hard to control with immunosuppressive drugs [7,30]. There may be a different HLA association [31].

Patients with late-onset MG (LOMG) are seldom thymectomised because they are thought not to benefit. The few thymic samples studied have shown only the normal age changes: fatty replacement of parenchymal tissue and scattered remnants of mainly medullary epithelium with sparse lymphocytes [32]. Nevertheless, some degree of thymopoiesis can persist even into the seventh decade [1, 47], presumably providing the substrate whence thymomas can grow in later life. Interestingly, about 30% of LOMG patients have auto-antibody profiles so similar to those typical in MG/thymoma patients [33] (Table 6.1) as to suggest that they might have rejected an occult thymoma after it had initiated their autoimmune responses.

Thymoma and MG

These uncommon and highly variable tumours have been studied intensively, largely because of their regular associations with certain autoimmune diseases/autoantibodies; for example, thymoma with MG is a classic paraneoplastic syndrome. The tumour is apparently involved in autoimmunisation, as in the Lambert-Eaton Myasthenic Syndrom (LEMS), though the mechanisms are less clear (see below). The resulting autoimmune disorders should be a valuable early warning sign of an underlying thymoma.

Around 30% of all thymoma patients develop MG [34]; about another 5% have pure red cell aplasia (PRCA), neutropenia, other bone marrow aplasias or hypogammaglobulinaemia that are again apparently autoimmune; associations with polymyositis have also been reported [35]. Uncomplicated thymomas tend to present late and sporadically, and have been studied much less.

The patient's myasthenia shows no obvious differences from the other subgroups`, except that it is almost always generalised (rather than pure ocular) and is always accompanied by anti-AChR rather than anti-MuSK antibodies [8]. It can be harder to treat, and it often worsens – or may even begin – after thymomectomy [36]. In general, its severity does not correlate with the tumour status, which therefore demands careful monitoring, even when the myasthenia is well controlled.

Certain other auto-antibodies are found in most thymoma patients with MG and in some without; they are also found in some LOMG patients who clearly have no thymoma, even at thymectomy or after prolonged follow-up (Table 6.1). Among the "anti-striated muscle auto-antibodies", those that recognise titin (found in >95% of MG/thymoma patients) or the ryanodine receptor (around 40%) are the best characterised [37, 38]. Surprisingly, neutralising auto-antibodies against all the subtypes of Interferon-α (>70%) and/or IL-12 (>50%) are also very prevalent at diagnosis [39]. Their striking increases around the time of thymoma recurrence (12 of 13 cases [40]) may be a valuable warning sign while patients are being monitored. They may also contribute to the occasional intractable infections in some patients, which are surprisingly rare, even in patients taking immunosuppressive drugs [21].

As reviewed incahpter 7, thymomas are neoplasms of thymic epithelial cells [41]. These show very heterogeneous cytogenetic changes [42]; they usually have a spindle cell (medullary) morphology in WHO types A and AB, both of which are nearly always benign [43, 44, 45]. In types B1–B3, the epithelial cells are typically plump/polygonal, and more often show more nuclear atypia in B3 than B2 and B1 (Table 6.2). In addition, maturing polyclonal thymocytes are abundant in types B1 and B2, which resemble disorganised cortex [46], and they are also very numerous in type AB; many of their progeny are clearly exported to the periphery [47]. Types B2 and especially B3 thymomas are often invasive. Further details are given in the legend for Table 6.2.

Pre-treatment with corticosteroids (for MG or PRCA) clearly can deplete the thymocytes moderately or drastically [46]. Thus, it can almost certainly change type AB histology towards type A, and type B1 towards B2; also B2 towards B3, so a B3 thymoma in a steroid-treated patient may not be as malignant as first appears. In fact, steroid pre-treatment can cause serious difficulties in interpretation, especially if the pathologist has not been informed of this.

For tumour prognosis, staging [48] was previously the most useful indicator [49], and should be carefully recorded at operation. The new WHO classification, however, now clearly adds independent prognostic value (Table 6.2) [44, 45, 50]; the prognosis is especially good with types A and AB, and even with types B1–B3 if removal has been complete and adjuvant therapy is given.

As will be described in Chap. 12, post-operative radiotherapy clearly reduces the risk of recurrence of invasive

Table 6.2 Thymoma Types

WHO type/ previous	immature thymocytes	% of all thymomas	% that develop MG	% that invade:		(%) 5 year survival
				ex capsule	further	
A spindle (medullary)	–	~10	10–20	~30	~10	100
AB mixed Type A + LE	++ to +++	~20	10–20	~30	~5	>80
B1 Organoid	++++	~10	~20	~25	~20	>80
B2 LE or cortical	++ to +++	~20	~40	~15	50–60	~80
B3 WDTC	+ to ++	~15	~30	~20	~60	~60
C Carcinoma	–	~20	<<5	~15	~50	~50

Recent sources: reviews by Chen et al (2002), Kim et al (2004), Kondo and Monden (2005) [44,45,50]

NB for the less common subtypes, the percentages are inevitably more approximate

B1, also called "predominantly cortical"; LE, lympho-epithelial

WDTC, well differentiated thymic carcinoma

Type A consists almost entirely of spindle (medullary) epithelial cells (often CD20+), with bland nuclear morphology. Frequently, they are arranged in a storiform (i.e. whorled) pattern, and lymphocytes are always rare

Type AB includes areas of type A mixed with lymphocyte-rich regions, where the epithelial cells often also have spindle morphology, but may appear more like type B2

Type B1 thymomas, like the others, clearly show the gross appearances of discrete tumours, but, microscopically, they may be hard to distinguish from normal thymus; hence the "organoid" label. They include large, clearly cortical areas; the occasional medullary foci even include Hassall's corpuscles

Type B2 consists of lobules of epithelial cells intimately mixed with immature thymocytes, which may be so abundant as to conceal the epithelial cells. These are usually oval or polygonal with vesicular nuclei, and frequently show a variable mixture of cortical and medullary markers, but often with weaker HLA-class II than in the normal cortex (46). Perivascular spaces are usually prominent and are frequently palisaded by epithelial cells

Type B3 consists mainly of round epithelial cells (often CD5+), but always with some immature thymocytes

The epithelial cells show nuclear atypia more often in B3 than B2 or B1

Type C includes carcinomas similar to those occurring elsewhere; they can be squamous, lympho-epitheliomatous, muco-epidermoid or undifferentiated

As discussed in the text, thymocyte depletion by corticosteroid pre-treatment (46) can almost certainly change type AB histology towards type A, type B1 towards B2, and type B2 towards B3

thymomas. Very aggressive tumours are commoner in younger subjects (<age 50), but can show surprisingly good responses to chemotherapy even at advanced stages [51, 52]. Although it associates more often with the more aggressive types B2 and B3, MG seems not to confer a worse tumour prognosis, probably because it also leads to earlier presentation [34]. Also, the steroids so often used may slow tumour growth [53].

The adjacent uninvolved thymus typically shows hyperplastic changes very similar to those in EOMG, especially in patients with MG [41]; since it may be involved in the autoimmunising process [54], it should be removed at the same time as the thymoma. However, the myasthenia seldom improves clearly after thymomectomy, and more often deteriorates.

Autoimmunising Mechanisms

Whereas type A thymomas are said to predominate in PRCA [55] and hypogammaglobulinaemia, MG most commonly associates with type B2 (Table 6.2). Some workers believe that generation of thymocytes in a disorganised pseudo-cortical B2 environment, often with reduced HLA-class II on the epithelial cells, leads to export of T cells that have never been properly screened for autoreactivity, and are therefore liable to initiate autoimmune responses in the periphery [56]. However, the almost exclusive associations with MG and bone marrow aplasias suggest a more specific bias in thymocyte selection or even active immunisation within the thymoma [54, 21]. Since myoid cells are rare or absent in thymomas, and intact AChR is undetectable [57], it seems most likely that the neoplastic epithelial cells autoimmunise T cells against isolated AChR subunits [58, 21] and that these initiate specific antibody responses after they have been exported. The apparent autoimmunisation against IFN-α (and IL-12) in thymomas as different as types A and B2 may implicate ubiquitous cell types such as dendritic cells or macrophages.

The management of MG has been reviewed by Vincent et al. [59], Palace et al. [60], Richman and Agius [61] and

Newsom-Davis [62]. Though it seldom improves MG, thymectomy is essential for most patients with thymoma (unless very frail) because of potential invasiveness. Most neurologists in Europe recommend thymectomy for anti-AChR⁺ patients with generalised MG that started before age 40 to 45 (or even 50), preferably as soon as they are fit for surgery. Its value in other subgroups is even less well established.

Differential Diagnoses

The rare congenital myasthenias are due to inherited defects in neuromuscular transmission, which are in no way immunological, so these patients do not benefit from thymectomy or immunosuppressive drugs. Neonatal MG is caused by passive transfer of anti-AChR autoantibodies from an MG mother to her baby. It normally wanes within a few weeks, never to return in later life. In rare cases where the mother has particularly pathogenic antibodies against the fetal AChR, there may be arthrogryposis multiplex congenita, with joint contractures, oesophageal or pulmonary malformations, or even perinatal death [63]. Juvenile MG (onset before puberty) is rare in Caucasians, but shows hints of differences from the other subgroups; the thymus is often normal, and our few patients show little sign of the HLA associations noted in other subgroups (Table 6.1).

Lambert-Eaton myasthenic syndrome (LEMS) is an important differential diagnosis of MG in adults, partly because the thymus is not involved, and thymectomy is not recommended. Among the characteristic clinical differences, the weakness predominantly affects the proximal limb muscles rather than those of the head and neck [11, 64]. Also, strength tends to increase with increasing effort, showing post-tetanic potentiation on EMG. LEMS is mediated by auto-antibodies [65] against voltage-gated calcium channels (VGCC) in motor nerve terminals that reduce ACh release [66]. Because these VGCC are similar in autonomic nerve endings, patients very often also have a dry mouth, constipation or impotence (in men), which are further valuable diagnostic clues. There is a highly sensitive and specific RIA for the anti-VGCC antibodies [67].

About 50% of patients have small cell lung cancer (SCLC), so LEMS is a classic paraneoplastic syndrome. SCLC cells express similar VGCC that apparently auto-immunise against those at the nerve terminals [68]. They evidently do so up to two years (or even more) before the tumour would otherwise be detected, so they clearly lead to earlier clinical presentation. Moreover, if the tumour can be removed or destroyed, the antibody levels tend to decline and the patient's has the strength to improve [69]. Interestingly, too, SCLC tumours sometimes grow more slowly in patients with LEMS, and there are occasional remarkably long-term survivors [70].

References

1. Sempowski G, Thomasch J, Gooding M, et al. Effect of thymectomy on human peripheral blood T cell pools in myasthenia gravis. J Immunol 2001;166:2808–2817.

2. Gill J, Malin M, Sutherland J, Gray D, Hollander G, Boyd R. Thymic generation and regeneration. Immunol Rev 2003;195:28–50.

3. Germain RN. T cell development and the CD4-CD8 lineage decision. Nat Rev Immunol 2002;2:309–322.

4. Sakaguchi S. Naturally arising Foxp3-expressing CD25+CD4+ regulatory T cells in immuno-logical tolerance to self and non-self. Nat Immunol 2005;6:345–352.

5. Newsom-Davis J, Beeson D. Myasthenia gravis and myasthenic syndromes. In Karpati G, Hilton-Jones D, Griggs R. Disorders of Voluntary Muscle, 7th edn. Cambridge University Press, 2001, pp 650–675.

6. Engel AG, Ohno K, Sine SM. Sleuthing molecular targets for neurological disease at the neuromuscular junction. Nat Rev Neurosci 2003;4:339–352.

7. Vincent A. Unravelling the pathogenesis of myasthenia gravis. Nat Rev Immunol 2002;2:797–804.

8. Vincent A, Drachman DB. Myasthenia gravis. Adv Neurol 2002;88:159–188.

9. Beeson D, Jacobson L, Newsom-Davis J, Vincent A. A transfected human muscle cell line expressing the adult subtype of the human muscle acetylcholine receptor for diagnostic assays in myasthenia gravis. Neurology 1996;47:1552–1555.

10. McConville J, Farrugia ME, Beeson D, et al. Detection and characterization of MuSK antibodies in seronegative myasthenia gravis. Ann Neurol 2004;55:580–584.

11. Wirtz PW, Sotodeh M, Nijnuis M, et al. Difference in distribution of muscle weakness between myasthenia gravis and the Lambert-Eaton myasthenic syndrome. J Neurol Neurosurg Psychiat 2002;73:766–768.

12. Kubo T, Noda M, Takai T, et al. Primary structure of delta subunit precursor of calf muscle acetylcholine receptor deduced from cDNA sequence. Eur J Biochem 1985;149:5–13.

13. Tzartos SJ, Barkas T, Cung MT, et al. Anatomy of the antigenic structure of a large membrane autoantigen, the muscle-type nicotinic acetylcholine receptor. Immunol Rev 1998;163:89–120.

14. Engel AG, Lambert EH, Howard FM. Immune complexes (IgG and C3) at the motor end-plate in myasthenia gravis: ultrastructural and light microscopic localization and electrophysiologic correlations. Mayo Clin Proc 1977;l52:267–280.

15. Hoch W, McConville J, Helms S, Newsom-Davis J, Melms A, Vincent A. Autoantibodies to the receptor tyrosine kinase MuSK in patients with myasthenia gravis without anti-acetylcholine receptor antibodies. Nature Medicine 2001;7:365–368.

16. Keynes G. History of myasthenia gravis. Med Hist 1961;5:313–326.

17. Jaretzki A, Steinglass KM and Sonett JR. Thymectomy in the management of myasthenia gravis. Semin Neurol 2004;24:49–62.

18. Gronseth GS, Barohn RJ. Practice parameter: thymectomy for myasthenia gravis (an evidence-based review). Neurology 2000;55:7–15.

19. Janer M, Cowland A, Picard J, et al. A susceptibility region for MG extending into the HLA-class I sector telomeric to HLA-C. Human Immunol 1999;60:909–917.

20. Roxanis I, Micklem K, Willcox N. Thymic myoid cells and germinal center formation in myasthenia gravis; possible roles in pathogenesis. J Neuroimmunol 2002;125:185–197.

21. Shiono H, Roxanis I, Zhang W, et al. Scenarios for autoimmunization of T and B cells in myasthenia gravis. Ann N Y Acad Sci 2003;998:237–256.

22. Meraouna A, Cizeron-Clairac G, Le Panse R, et al. The chemokine CXCL13 is a key molecule in autoimmune Myasthenia Gravis. Blood prepublished online March 16, 2006; DOI 10.1182/blood-2005-06-2383.

23. Schluep M, Willcox N, Vincent A, Dhoot GK, Newsom-Davis J. Acetylcholine receptors in human thymic myoid cells in situ: an immunohistological study. Ann Neurol 1987;22:212–222.

24. McHeyzer-Williams LJ, McHeyzer-Williams MG. Antigen-specific memory B cell development. Annu Rev Immunol 2005;23:487–513.

25. Matthews I, Sims GP, Ledwidge S, Stott DI, Willcox N, Vincent A. Antibodies to human acetylcholine receptor in parous women: evidence for immunization by fetal antigen. Lab Invest 2002;82:1407–1417.

26. Willcox HN, Newsom-Davis J, Calder LR. Greatly increased autoantibody production in myasthenia gravis by thymocyte suspensions prepared with proteolytic enzymes. Clin Exp Immunol 1983;54:378–386.

27. Willcox N, Schluep M, Sommer N, et al. Variable corticosteroid sensitivity of thymic cortex and medullary peripheral-type lymphoid tissue in myasthenia gravis patients: structural and functional effects. Quart J Med 1989;73:1071–1087.

28. Leite MI, Strobel P, Jones M, et al. Fewer thymic changes in MuSK antibody-positive than in MuSK antibody-negative MG. Ann Neurol 2005;57:444–448.

29. Lauriola L, Ranelletti F, Maggiano N, et al. Thymus changes in anti-MuSK-positive and -negative myasthenia gravis. Neurology 2005;64:536–538.

30. Evoli A, Tonali PA, Padua L. Clinical correlates with anti-MuSK antibodies in generalized seronegative myasthenia gravis. Brain 2003;126:2304–2311.

31. Niks EH, Kuks JB, Roep BO, et al. Strong association of MuSK antibody-positive myasthenia gravis and HLA-DR14-DQ5. Neurology 2006;66:1772–1774.

32. Steinmann GG, Klaus B, Muller-Hermelink HK. The involution of the ageing human thymic epithelium is independent of puberty: a morphometric study. Scand J Immunol 1985;22:563–575.

33. Giraud M, Beaurain G, Yamamoto AM, et al. Linkage of HLA to myasthenia gravis and genetic heterogeneity depending on anti-titin antibodies. Neurology 2001;57:1555–1560.

34. Kondo K, Monden Y. Thymoma and myasthenia gravis: a clinical study of 1,089 patients from Japan. Ann Thorac Surg 2005;79:219–224.

35. Souadjian JV, Enriquez P, Silverstein MN, Pepin JM. The spectrum of diseases associated with thymoma: coincidence or syndrome? Arch Int Med 1974;134:374–379.

36. Namba T, Brunner NG, Grob D. Myasthenia gravis in patients with thymoma, with particular reference to onset after thymectomy. Medicine (Baltimore) 1978;57:411–433.

37. Aarli JA, Stefansson K, Marton LS, Wollmann RL. Patients with myasthenia gravis and thymoma have in their sera IgG autoantibodies against titin. Clin Exp Immunol 1990;82:284–288.

38. Mygland A, Tysnes OB, Matre R, Volpe P, Aarli JA, Gilhus NE. Ryanodine receptor autoantibodies in myasthenia gravis patients with a thymoma. Ann Neurol 1992;32:589–591.

39. Meager A, Wadhwa M, Dilger P, et al. Anti-cytokine autoantibodies in autoimmunity: preponderance of neutralizing autoantibodies against interferon-alpha, interferon-omega and interleukin-12 in patients with thymoma and/or myasthenia gravis. Clin Exp Immunol 2003;132:128–136.

40. Buckley C, Newsom-Davis J, Willcox N, Vincent A. Do titin and cytokine antibodies in MG patients predict thymoma or thymoma recurrence? Neurology 2001;57:1579–1582.

41. Rosai J, Levine GD. Tumors of the thymus. In Atlas of tumor pathology. US Armed Forces Institute of Pathology, Washington, DC, 1976, 2nd Series, Fascicle 13.

42. Inoue M, Starostik P, Zettl A, et al. Correlating genetic aberrations with World Health Organization-defined histology and stage across the spectrum of thymomas. Cancer Res 2003;63:3708–3715.

43. Marx A, Müller-Hermelink H. From basic immunobiology to the upcoming WHO-classification of tumors and the thymus. Path Res Practice 1999;195:515–533.

44. Chen G, Marx A, Wen-Hu C, et al. New WHO histologic classification predicts prognosis of thymic epithelial tumors: a clinicopathologic study of 200 thymoma cases from China. Cancer 2002;95:420–429.

45. Kim DJ, Yang WI, Choi SS, Kim KD, Chung KY. Prognostic and clinical relevance of the World Health Organization schema for the classification of thymic epithelial tumors: a clinicopathologic study of 108 patients and literature review. Chest 2005;127:755–761.

46. Willcox N, Schluep M, Ritter MA, Schuurman HJ, Newsom-Davis J, Christensson B. Myasthenic and nonmyasthenic thymoma. An expansion of a minor cortical epithelial cell subset? Am J Pathol 1987;127:447–460.

47. Buckley C, Douek D, Newsom-Davis J, Vincent A, Willcox N. Mature, long-lived CD4+ and CD8+ T cells are generated by thymomas in myasthenia gravis. Ann Neurol 2001;50:64–72.

48. Masaoka A, Monden Y, Nakahara K, Tanioka T. Follow-up study of thymomas with special reference to their clinical stages. Cancer 1981;48:2485–2492.

49. Verley JM, Hollmann KH. Thymoma. A comparative study of clinical stages, histologic features, and survival in 200 cases. Cancer 1985;55:1074–1086.

50. Kondo K, Yoshizawa K, Tsuyuguchi M, et al. WHO histologic classification is a prognostic indicator in thymoma. Ann Thorac Surg 2004;77:1183–1188.

51. Kesler KA, Wright CD, Loehrer PJ. Thymoma: current medical and surgical management. Semin Neurol 2004;24:63–73.

52. Giaccone G. Treatment of malignant thymoma. Curr Opin Oncol 2005;17:140–146.

53. Loehrer PJ Sr, Wang W, Johnson DH, Aisner SC, Ettinger DS. Octreotide alone or with prednisone in patients with advanced thymoma and thymic carcinoma: an Eastern Cooperative Oncology Group Phase II Trial. J Clin Oncol 2004;22:293–299.

54. Willcox N. Myasthenia gravis. Curr Opin Immunol 1993;5:910–917.

55. Kuo T, Shih LY. Histologic types of thymoma associated with pure red cell aplasia: a study of five cases including a composite tumor of organoid thymoma associated with an unusual lipofibroadenoma. Int J Surg Pathol 2001;9:29–35.

56. Kadota Y, Okumura M, Miyoshi S, et al. Altered T cell development in human thymoma is related to impairment of MHC class II transactivator expression induced by interferon-gamma (IFN-gamma). Clin Exp Immunol 2000;121:59–68.

57. Siara J, Rudel R, Marx A. Absence of acetylcholine-induced current in epithelial cells from thymus glands and thymomas of myasthenia gravis patients. Neurology 1991;41:128–131.

58. Nagvekar N, Moody AM, Moss P, et al. A pathogenetic rôle for the thymoma in myasthenia gravis; autosensitization of IL4-producing T cell clones recognising extracellular AChR epitopes presented by minority class II isotypes. J Clin Invest 1998;101:2268–2277.

59. Vincent A, Palace J and Hilton-Jones D. Myasthenia gravis. Lancet 2001;357:212–218.

60. Palace J, Vincent A, Beeson D. Myasthenia gravis: diagnostic and management dilemmas. Curr Opin Neurol 2001;14:583–589.

61. Richman DP, Agius M. Treatment of autoimmune myasthenia gravis. Neurology 2003;61:1652–1661.

62. Newsom-Davis J. Therapy in MG and Lambert-Eaton myasthenic syndrome. Semin Neurol 2003;23:191–198.

63. Riemersma S, Vincent A, Beeson D, et al. Association of arthrogryposis multiplex congenita with maternal antibodies inhibiting fetal acetylcholine receptor function. J Clin Invest 1996;98:2358–2363.

64. O' Neill JH, Murray NM, Newsom-Davis J. The Lambert-Eaton myasthenic syndrome. A review of 50 cases. Brain 1988;111:577–596.

65. Lang B, Newsom-Davis J, Wray D, Vincent A and Murray N. Autoimmune aetiology for the myasthenic (Eaton-Lambert) syndrome. Lancet 1981;2:224–226.

66. Pinto A, Iwasa K, Newland C, Newsom-Davis J, Lang B. The action of Lambert-Eaton myasthenic syndrome immunoglobulin G on cloned human voltage–gated calcium channels. Muscle & Nerve 2002;25:715–724.

67. Motomura M, Johnston I, Lang B, Vincent A, Newsom-Davis J. An improved diagnostic assay for Lambert-Eaton myasthenic syndrome. J Neurol Neurosurg Psychiat 1995;58:85–87.

68. Roberts A, Perera S, Lang B, Vincent A, Newsom-Davis J. Paraneoplastic myasthenic syndrome IgG inhibits 45Ca2+ flux in a human small cell carcinoma line. Nature 1985;317:737–739.

69. Chalk CH, Murray NM, Newsom-Davis J, O' Neill JH, Spiro SG. Response of the Lambert-Eaton myasthenic syndrome to treatment of associated small-cell lung carcinoma. Neurology 1990;40:1552–1556.

70. Maddison P, Newsom-Davis J, Mills KR, Souhami, RL Favourable prognosis in the Lambert-Eaton myasthenic syndrome and small cell lung carcinoma. Lancet 1999;353:117–118.

Surgical Pathology

7

Elizabeth Soilleux and Colin Clelland

Introduction

As a result of the complicated embryological development of the thymus, and its complex structure and function, a wide range of thymic pathology is possible – although many such pathological changes are rare. Pathology in the thymus can be divided up into thymic cysts, hyperplasia and tumours. Neuroendocrine tumours, germ cell tumours and haematopoietic tumours are comparatively rare, while thymomas and thymic carcinomas are more common. Biopsies, or occasionally frozen sections, may be used to determine whether a particular lesion requires excision. Cysts, symptomatic hyperplasia and thymic tumours, with the exception of lymphomas, seminomas and malignant non-seminomatous germ cell tumours, usually require excision.

The Importance of Thymic Surgical Pathology

A number of conditions can lead to thymic enlargement. The thymus may be biopsied to determine the cause of the enlargement, or excised as a primary treatment or to relieve compression of adjacent structures. Recent experience in Oxford in thymic surgical pathology is summarised in Table 7.1. Thymic biopsies are usually performed to determine whether thymectomy is required. With the exception of lymphomas and some germ cell tumours, a diagnosis of neoplasia within the thymus generally leads to thymectomy [1, 2], while non-neoplastic conditions, such as hyperplasia, will only lead to thymic excision if associated with other symptoms, such as those of myasthenia gravis [2].

Specimen Examination in Thymic Surgical Pathology

The majority of specimens will be placed in neutral buffered formalin (NBF) at the time of excision. However, occasionally an intra-operative diagnosis may be required; for example, if there are unexpected findings in or closely related to the thymus. Accordingly, a small piece of tissue will be sent to the laboratory for frozen section. While this often results in a diagnosis, there may be difficulties in distinguishing lymphoma from small cell carcinoma and poorly differentiated squamous cell carcinoma. Lymphoma may also be difficult to distinguish from thymic hyperplasia [3].

For excision specimens, the macroscopic appearance is described and the specimen weighed, following removal of fat if necessary. In addition to the sampling of surgical resection margins, particular attention is paid to representative sampling of each area with a different macroscopic appearance. Ink may be applied to surgical resection margins in order to permit microscopic evaluation for involvement by tumour. Sections for histological examination are generally available two to three days post-operatively.

Table 7.1 Audit of surgical thymic pathology in Oxford from 1983 to 2002

Normal	Thymoma	Thymic carcinoma	Carcinoid	Lymphoma*	Cyst	Involution
63 (28)	63 (28)	13 (5.5)	2 (1)	5 (2)	8 (3.5)	11 (5)

Number (percentage) of each diagnostic category of 226 cases.
* four non-Hodgkin's lymphomas and one Hodgkin's disease

Classification of Thymic Pathology

The major causes of thymic enlargement are cysts, hyperplasia and neoplasms [2, 4]. Cysts may be congenital or acquired, with the latter having a greater risk of being associated with inflammation and neoplasms, such as thymoma, thymic carcinoma and Hodgkin's lymphoma [2, 4]. Thymic hyperplasia is important for two reasons. First, it should be distinguished from thymic neoplasia, particularly thymomas; and second, it may be associated with autoimmune conditions, including myasthenia gravis and rheumatoid arthritis [2]. Neoplasms in the thymus may be divided up in a number of ways [2, 4]. The vast majority are primary, as metastases to the thymus are very rare. Primary tumours can be considered in terms of whether they show differentiation towards intrinsic thymic tissues, such as epithelium, lymphoid tissue and stroma, or differentiation towards other tissue types, such as neuroendocrine and germ cell tumours (Fig. 7.1). The exact histogenesis of neuroendocrine and germ cell tumours remains uncertain. Table 7.2 gives an overview of lesions arising in the thymus, and is derived from the WHO classification [4, 5]. Rarely, thymic tumours or tumour-like lesions defy classification. Neoplasms may arise in ectopic thymic tissue, which is found in areas embryologically related to the branchial pouches, such as the neck and mediastinum, e.g. an ectopic hamartomatous thymoma [2]. Further details of these tumours can be found in standard surgical pathology texts.

Pathology of Lesions Arising in the Thymus

Cysts

Cysts are fluid filled spaces that are lined by epithelium. Thymic cysts are rare, and the majority – particularly those that are unilocular – are believed to be congenital in origin. The acquired cysts may be associated with other pathology, such as Hodgkin's and non-Hodgkin's lymphomas and HIV infection, or may be reactive in origin, for example in inflammatory processes [2, 4]. True thymic cysts must be separated from other cystic lesions, including cystic thymoma, cystic teratoma, lymphangioma, mediastinal cysts and cystic change in other lesions (Fig. 7.2), as the latter may carry a different prognosis [2]. Macroscopically, cysts appear round or oval and uni- or multiloculated, with thin walls and attached fatty thymic tissue. The contents range from clear, colourless fluid to straw-coloured to chocolate coloured when previous haemorrhage has occurred. Histologically, cysts may be lined by flattened, cuboidal, columnar, respiratory-type or stratified squamous epithelium, some or part of which

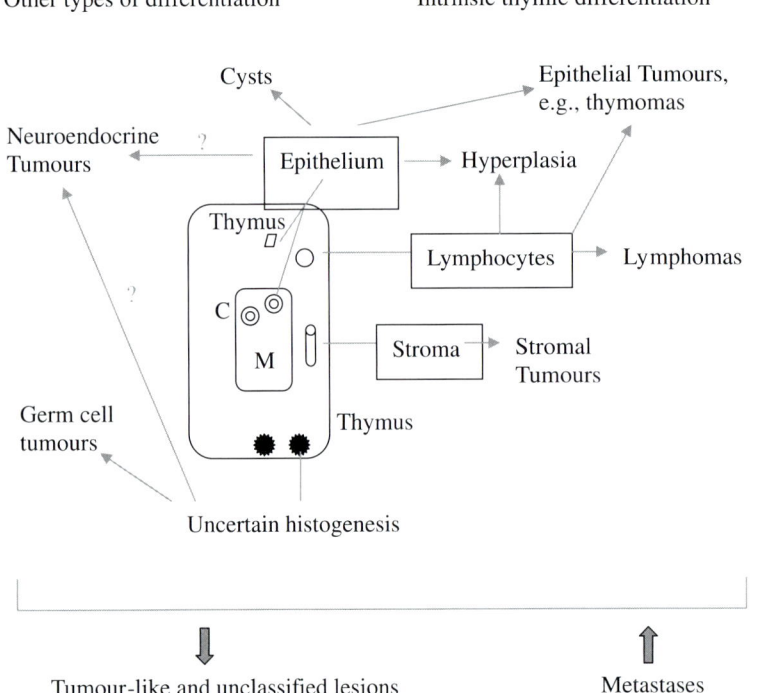

Fig. 7.1 Summary of types of pathological conditions arising in the thymus (*C*, cortex; *M*, medulla)

Table 7.2 Summary of main types of surgical pathology arising in the thymus

Cysts	Congenital (often unilocular) Acquired (often multilocular and may be associated with neoplasms)
Hyperplasia	True thymic hyperplasia (associated with myasthenia gravis) Lymphoid hyperplasia (associated with other autoimmune conditions)
Thymomas	Divided into types A, AB, B1, B2 and B3 on basis of numbers of lymphocytes and appearances of epithelial cells (WHO Classification, 1999)
Thymic carcinoma	Various different types of epithelial differentiation possible
Haematopoietic neoplasms	B cell non-Hodgkin's lymphoma Hodgkin's lymphoma T cell lymphoma Langerhans cell histiocytosis
Stromal Tumours	Thymolipoma Thymoliposarcoma Rhabdoid tumour Localised fibrous tumour
Germ Cell Tumours	Mature Teratoma Seminoma/germinoma Malignant non-seminomatous germ cell tumour
Neuroendocrine	Typical carcinoids Atypical carcinoids Large cell neuroendocrine tumours Small cell carcinoma

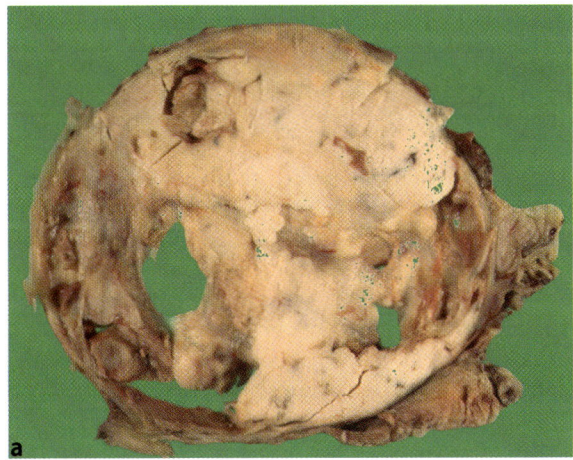
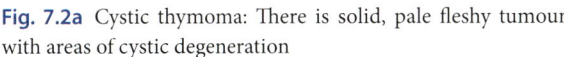
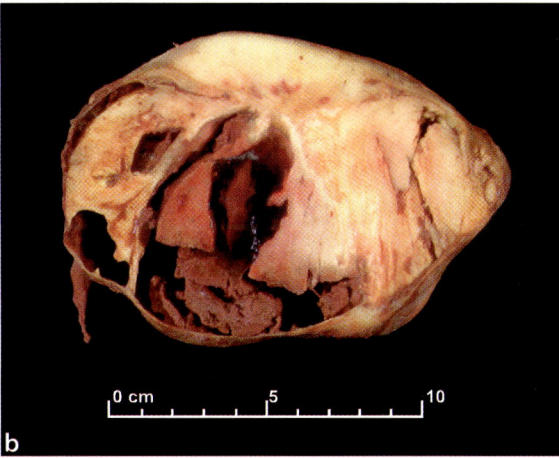

Fig. 7.2a Cystic thymoma: There is solid, pale fleshy tumour with areas of cystic degeneration

Fig. 7.2b Thymolipoma: There is significant haemorrhage in several areas resulting in a cystic appearance

may have been replaced by granulation tissue due to the pressure of the fluid within the cyst. Carcinoma of the lining epithelium occurs, but is rare [2].

Hyperplasia

Hyperplasia in the thymus is defined in two ways. True thymic hyperplasia refers to an increase in normally organised thymic tissue, as determined by comparing the weight of the explanted thymus with standard weight charts [6]. Lymphoid hyperplasia refers to the presence of increased numbers of lymphoid follicles and germinal centres within the thymus, and is rarely associated with an increase in the size of the gland [2]. However, in contrast to thymoma, the macroscopically visible configuration of the thymus gland is preserved in both types of thymic hyperplasia [2]. Although the number of lymphoid follicles required to diagnose lymphoid hyperplasia is not well defined, conspicuous numbers of follicles would attract a diagnosis of lymphoid hyperplasia [2]. However, in the normal thymus, small numbers of lymphoid follicles are seen at the cortico-medullary junction [7]. Lymphoid hyperplasia is most commonly associated with myasthenia gravis, but may occur in the setting of other autoimmune processes, including systemic lupus erythematosus, rheumatoid arthritis, scleroderma, vasculitis and autoimmune thyroid disorders [2].

Thymomas

Thymomas are usually encapsulated tumours that, in contrast to hyperplasia, distort the normal gross configuration of the thymus [2, 4]. Macroscopically, they appear fleshy and are often traversed by fibrous bands. Invasion through the capsule and possibly into adjacent structures may be seen in widely invasive thymomas. The neoplastic cells of thymomas show morphological and immunohistochemical features of thymic epithelial cells, with or without an admixed population of small T-lymphocytes. If clear-cut atypia of the epithelial cells is present, the tumour is classified as a thymic carcinoma [2, 4]. Various morphological subclassifications of thymomas exist, but here we will use the WHO classification (1999) and compare it with the previously widely used Muller-Hermelink classification [4, 8] (Fig. 7.3). The morphological features of a thymoma are usually adequate to avoid misdiagnoses, which include anterior mediastinal lymph nodes, lymphoma, seminoma and carcinoid tumour. When there is difficulty, cytokeratin immunostaining may be undertaken to demonstrate the epithelial component of the thymoma [9]. Depending on the relative ratios of epithelium and lymphocytes, and on the part of thymus that they recapitulate most closely, thymomas

are classified into five major subtypes (Table 7.3) [4, 8]. In thymomas at less advanced stages, morphological subtype plays a role in the prediction of prognosis, with types A and AB predicting improved survival [8, 10]. Although thymomas (particularly types A and AB (Table 7.3) are not categorised as malignant, because they do not show definite atypia, even thymomas with very bland histological features may metastasise. As with most tumours that have the potential to metastasise, tumour staging is an important predictor of prognosis [11]. Staging of thymomas, using the Masaoka system, in addition to stage-related prognosis, is summarised in Table 7.4 [4, 11].

Thymic Carcinoma

Thymic carcinomas show overt features of malignancy, and frequently demonstrate foci of necrosis. They are cytokeratin-positive epithelial neoplasms that arise in the thymus and that show overt cytological features of malignancy [4]. They may show some features suggesting differentiation towards a thymic epithelial phenotype, but a wide range of appearances analogous to various carcinomas seen at other sites, e.g. squamous cell carcinoma, is also possible [4]. Staging of thymic carcinomas also relies on the Masaoka staging system (Table 7.4) [4].

Haematopoietic Disorders

The major haematopoietic disorders occurring in the thymus are summarised in Table 7.5 [4,5].

Stromal Tumours

Thymolipomas are composed of islands of microscopically unremarkable thymic parenchyma interspersed with mature adipose tissue. They can cause massive thymic enlargement, often with retention of the normal gross configuration of the thymus, but show benign behaviour [2]. The cut surface of a thymolipoma is yellow and lobulated, similar to that of a lipoma, but small white streaks and nodules of thymic tissue are also present [2] (Fig. 7.2b). Thymolipomas may be associated with similar conditions to those associated with true thymic hyperplasia, such as myasthenia gravis [2].

Thymoliposarcomas are very rare malignant liposarcomas that infiltrate the thymus, entrapping thymic tissue and exhibiting an intimate anatomical relationship with thymic stroma [4, 13]. Macroscopically, the tumour may be a large grey mass, which may appear surprisingly well circumscribed [14].

Localised (solitary) fibrous tumour (LFT) is a mesenchymal tumour of probable mesothelial histogenesis, which is composed of spindle cells with a fibroblastic

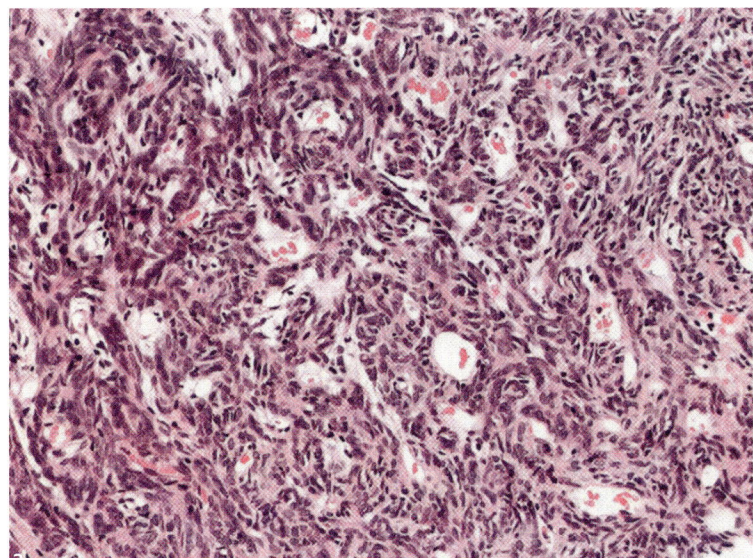

Fig. 7.3a Thymoma: WHO type A, medullary type by Muller-Hermelink classification. Bland spindle-shaped epithelial cells with few interspersed lymphocytes

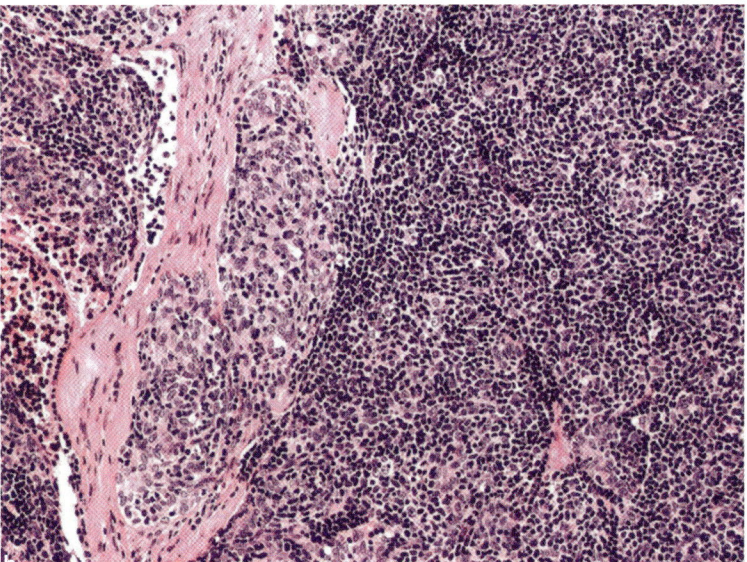

Fig. 7.3b Thymoma: WHO type B2, cortical type (recurrent) by Muller-Hermelink classification. Plump polygonal epithelial cells with prominent nucleoli outnumbered by immature lymphocytes

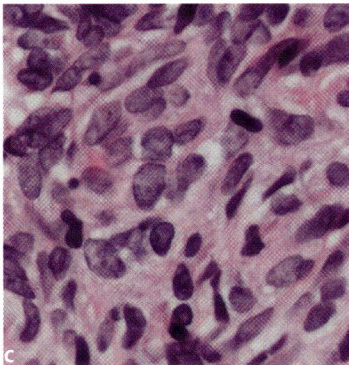

Fig. 7.3c High magnification of **3a** to show detail of bland spindle-shaped epithelial cells

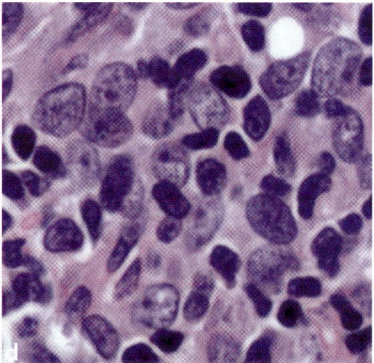

Fig. 7.3d High magnification of **3b** to show prominent nucleoli and granular chromatin pattern

Table 7.3 Features of the morphological subtypes of thymomas [4,8]

WHO Type	Müller-Hermelink Type/ Histogenetic differentiation	Morphology	10 year survival (%) [12]
A	Medullary thymoma	Round or oval neoplastic thymic epithelial cells, accompanied by few or no reactive lymphocytes. Epithelial cells show no nuclear atypia	100
AB	Mixed thymoma	Variably segregated areas show features of type A thymoma and type B thymoma	75
B1	Predominantly cortical (organoid)	Tumours almost exactly resemble normal thymic cortex with occasional areas of medullary differentiation, being composed of abundant non-atypical epithelial cells with lymphocytes present	92
B2	Cortical	Tumours resemble normal thymic cortex with more numerous epithelial cells than in B1. Epithelial cells also have larger nuclei and more conspicuous nucleoli	87.5
B3	Well differentiated thymic carcinoma	The tumour is composed of sheets of round or polygonal epithelial cells showing mild atypia, with few admixed lymphocytes	30
C	Thymic carcinoma (see below)	Epithelial cells show overt cytological features of malignancy	0 (for endocrine carcinomas)

Table 7.4 Masaoka staging system for thymomas and thymic carcinomas [4,11]

Stage	Histopathological findings	Simpler staging system	10 year survival (%)[11]
Stage I	Macroscopically encapsulated with no microscopically visible capsular invasion	Encapsulated	91–100
Stage II	Macroscopic invasion of mediastinal fatty tissue or mediastinal pleura, or microscopic invasion into the capsule	Minimally invasive	89–100
Stage III	Macroscopic invasion into surrounding structures (pericardium, great vessels, lung)	Widely invasive	47–60
Stage IV	A, pleural or pericardial dissemination; B, lymphatic or haematogenous metastases	Widely invasive	0–11

Table 7.5 Haematological disorders arising in the thymus [4,5]

Haematological disorder	Type of disorder	Morphology
Marginal zone lymphoma of mucosal-associated lymphoid tissue (MALT) type	Low grade B cell (CD20+, CD79a+) non-Hodgkin's lymphoma	Small lymphocytes and plasma cells with germinal centre formation
Diffuse large B cell lymphoma of thymic type	High grade B cell (CD20+, CD79a+) non-Hodgkin's lymphoma	Large, pleomorphic, atypical lymphocytes with a variably fibrotic background
Hodgkin's lymphoma (usually nodular sclerosing type)	Lymphoma composed of CD30+, CD15+ B-cells (Reed-Sternberg (RS) cells) with a background of mixed leucocytes	Nodular proliferation (numerous collagen bands present) comprising RS cells (possessing at least two large rounded nuclear lobes with prominent nucleoli in small lacunae, with admixed non-neoplastic small lymphocytes and eosinophils. Multiloculated cysts are frequently associated [2]
Lymphoblastic lymphoma	T cell-expressing TdT (a marker of differentiating lymphocytes)	Small- to medium-sized blastic lymphocytes some with convoluted nuclei
Langerhan's cell histiocytosis (LCH)	Clonal proliferation of CD1a+ antigen presenting Langerhan's cells.	Large Langerhan's cells with vesicular nuclei and nuclear grooves admixed with variable numbers of lymphocytes and eosinophils. LCH may lead to the development of thymic cysts

appearance, forming hyper- and hypocellular areas separated by dense keloidal collagen [4,15]. It can occur within the thymus and entrap thymic parenchyma. Macroscopically, it appears as a well circumscribed, sometimes partially encapsulated mass, with a multinodular, firm, white cut surface [15]. A small proportion of LFTs is associated with hypoglycaemia [15]. While the majority of LFTs are benign tumours cured by complete excision, a small proportion show malignant behaviour. The latter usually demonstrate some of the following histological features: increased mitotic activity, atypia, foci of necrosis and infiltrative margins [4, 15].

Rhabdoid tumours are rare, highly malignant tumours, which are densely cellular and are composed of sheets of small oval to round cells, the cytoplasm of which appears filled with hyaline, eosinophilic material, which displaces the nucleus to the periphery of the cell [4, 16].

Germ Cell Tumours

Thymic germ cell tumours are believed to develop from germ cells that have migrated to this extragonadal site during embryogenesis. The thymus is the most common site at which germ cell tumours develop within the mediastinum [4]. Thymic germ cell tumours occur in children and younger adults, and may be discovered incidentally or may present with symptoms of compression or with constitutional symptoms. Non-seminomatous germ cell tumours may also produce endocrine effects due to the production of β-human chorionic gonadotropin (β-hCG).

Pre-operatively, increased serum levels of β-hCG and/or alpha-fetoprotein (AFP) may be measurable in non-seminomatous germ cell tumours, while seminomas can lead to increased serum lactate dehydrogenase (LDH) [1, 2]. In diagnosing a thymic germ cell tumour, it is important to exclude a metastasis from a gonadal primary tumour by, for example, examination of the testes [17].

Thymic germ cell tumours are classified by their histological type, in a manner entirely analogous to gonadal germ cell tumours. Thymic germ cell tumours are divided into mature teratomas (which require surgical excision only and have a good prognosis), seminomas (which respond well to chemotherapy and radiotherapy) and malignant non-seminomatous germ cell tumours (MNS-GCTs) (which tend to have a poorer prognosis regardless of the modality of therapy used) [1]. The majority of thymic germ cell tumours are benign teratomas that have a good prognosis and are best treated with surgical excision, although malignant teratomas can also occur. Seminomas (analogous to the female germ cell tumours, dysgerminomas), the second most frequent thymic germ cell tumour, occur almost exclusively in males [1]. As in the testis, they may be associated with a dense inflammatory infiltrate, which may lead to the development of reactive multilocular thymic cysts [2].

Macroscopically, benign teratomas are encapsulated and generally predominantly cystic, often with fibrous adhesions to surrounding structures. Brown or oily fluid is often present and hair may be seen [2]. Most other thymic germ cell tumours are large, solid tumours that may adhere to or invade adjacent structures. Their cut surfaces

Table 7.6 Microscopic features of teratomas

Type of germ cell tumour	Microscopic findings	Approximate 5 year survival with current treatments [18]
Mature teratoma (and immature teratoma)	Tumour composed of benign, well differentiated (mature) or embryonic/fetal (immature) tissues derived from two or three germ layers (endoderm, mesoderm and ectoderm). Skin and its appendages, bronchial tissue, gastrointestinal mucosa, smooth muscle and fat are most frequently present [2]	76%
Seminoma (dys)germinoma	Sheets of large polygonal placental alkaline phosphatase (PLAP)+ cells with a distinct cell membrane, often with a prominent lymphocytic infiltrate	100%
Malignant non-seminomatous germ cell tumour (MNSGCT)	This may contain elements of immature teratoma, foci of seminoma, AFP+ areas with features of yolk sac differentiation, areas with features of β-HCG+ choriocarcinoma and very undifferentiated areas of cytokeratin+ embryonal carcinoma [2]	20%

Table 7.7 Thymic neuroendocrine tumours

Type of neuroendocrine tumour	Histological features
Typical carcinoid	A well differentiated tumour composed of uniform cells with neuroendocrine features [4]. Mitotic activity is scant and necrosis absent [4]
Atypical carcinoid	Architectural and cytological features are very similar to those of typical carcinoids. However, atypical carcinoids show increased mitotic activity (2–10 mitotic figures/mm^2) and/or punctate foci of necrosis [4]
Large cell neuroendocrine carcinoma	Features are similar to those of atypical carcinoid, except for the presence of much larger foci of necrosis and an increased mitotic rate (>10 mitotic figures/mm^2) [4]
Small cell carcinoma	Foci of necrosis and sheets of short spindle cells, with scant cytoplasm and ill-defined cell borders often demonstrating nuclear moulding [2, 22]

show a highly variable colour and texture, often with foci of haemorrhage and necrosis [1, 2]. Microscopic features are summarised in Table 7.6.

Tumours with Neuroendocrine Features

Using similar criteria to those used in the lung, thymic neuroendocrine tumours are classified as shown in Table 7.7 [4]. Typical carcinoids may be found incidentally or may present as a mass, or more rarely due to their endocrine activity, particularly ACTH production [2]. Some thymic carcinoids are associated with multiple endocrine neoplasia [2]. Macroscopically, carcinoids are variably sized, encapsulated or circumscribed tumours, with pale tan to grey white cut surfaces [2]. Small, scattered foci of necrosis or haemorrhage may be present in atypical carcinoid tumours. Carcinoids may adhere to or invade surrounding structures [2]. Although few studies have been performed, due to the rarity of thymic neuroendocrine tumours, it appears that the prognosis is relatively poor, even for well differentiated tumours [19–21].

Large cell neuroendocrine carcinoma and small cell carcinoma are both rare primary lesions in the thymus, but are not uncommon as metastatic mediastinel lesions from a lung cancer. They show similar histological features to the corresponding lung tumours (Table 7.7) [2, 4]. Their modes of presentation are similar to those of carcinoids [2] and macroscopically analogous to lung tumours; their microscopic appearances include larger foci of necrosis than carcinoids [19, 22]. Neuroendocrine tumours stain positively for some or all of the following markers: synaptophysin, chromogranin, pgp9.5 and CD56 [2, 4]. Thyroid transcription factor (TTF-1), a good marker for neoplasms of pulmonary origin, should be negative to differentiate a thymic metastasis from a pulmonary primary [23].

Metastatic Neoplasms

The thymus is most commonly involved by direct spread of neoplasms originating in other organs, particularly carcinoma of the lung. Pulmonary squamous and large cell carcinomas may be difficult to distinguish from thymic carcinoma, and a recent study shows that expression of TTF-1 by the tumour points to a lung primary, while CD5 expression by tumour cells and CD1a expression by infiltrating lymphocytes favour a thymic origin [24]. Haematogenous spread of neoplasms to the thymus is rare [4].

References

1. Strollo DC, Rosado-de-Christenson ML. Tumors of the thymus. J Thorac Imaging 1999;14:152–171.

2. Shimosato Y, Mukai K. Tumors of the mediastinum. In: Atlas of tumor pathology. Third series, 1997, Washington DC: Armed Forces Institute of Pathology under the auspices of Universities Associated for Research and Education in Pathology, p. 278.

3. Juttner FM, Fellbaum C, Popper H, Arian K, Pinter H, Friehs G. Pitfalls in intraoperative frozen section histology of mediastinal neoplasms. Eur J Cardiothorac Surg 1990;4:584–586.

4. Rosai J, Sobin LH, and World Health Organization. Histological typing of tumours of the thymus. In: International histological classification of tumours, 1999, Berlin: Springer. X, p. 65.

5. Jaffe ES and International Agency for Research on Cancer. Pathology and genetics of tumours of haematopoietic and lymphoid tissues. In: World Health Organization classification of tumours, 2001, Lyon: IARC Press, p. 351.

6. Steinmann GG, Klaus B, Muller-Hermelink HK. The involution of the ageing human thymic epithelium is independent of puberty. A morphometric study. Scand J Immunol 1985;22:563–575.

7. Middleton G, Schoch EM. The prevalence and age distribution of human thymic B lymphoid follicles. Pathology 1998;30:160–163.

8. Kirchner T, Schalke B, Marx A, Muller-Hermelink HK. Evaluation of prognostic features in thymic epithelial tumors. Thymus 1989;14:195–203.

9. Battifora H, Sun TT, Bahu RM, Rao S. The use of antikeratin antiserum as a diagnostic tool: thymoma versus lymphoma. Hum Pathol 1980;11:635–641.

10. Chen G, Marx A, Wen-Hu C, et al. New WHO histologic classification predicts prognosis of thymic epithelial tumors: a clinicopathologic study of 200 thymoma cases from China. Cancer 2002;95:420–429.

11. Johnson SB, Eng TY, Giaccone G, Thomas CR Jr. Thymoma: update for the new millennium. Oncologist 2001;6:239–246.

12. Lardinois D, Rechsteiner R, Lang RH, et al. Prognostic relevance of Masaoka and Muller-Hermelink classification in patients with thymic tumors. Ann Thorac Surg 2000;69:1550–1555.

13. Klimstra DS, Moran CA, Perino G, Koss MN, Rosai J. Liposarcoma of the anterior mediastinum and thymus. A clinicopathologic study of 28 cases. Am J Surg Pathol 1995;19:782–791.

14. Sung MT, Ko SF, Hsieh MJ, Chen YJ, Chen WJ, Huang HY. Thymoliposarcoma. Ann Thorac Surg 2003;76:2082–2085.

15. Fletcher CDM, Unni KK, Mertens F. Pathology and genetics of tumours of soft tissue and bone. In: World Health Organization classification of tumours, 2002, Lyon: IARC Press, p. 427.

16. Tamboli P, Toprani TH, Amin MB, et al. Carcinoma of lung with rhabdoid features. Hum Pathol 2004;35:8–13.

17. Suzuki K, Kurokawa K, Suzuki T, et al. Anterior mediastinal metastasis of testicular germ cell tumor: relation to benign thymic hyperplasia. Eur Urol 1997;32:371–374.

18. Takeda S, Miyoshi S, Ohta M, Minami M, Masaoka A, Matsuda H. Primary germ cell tumors in the mediastinum: a 50–year experience at a single Japanese institution. Cancer 2003;97:367–376.

19. Moran CA, Suster S. Thymic neuroendocrine carcinomas with combined features ranging from well-differentiated (carcinoid) to small cell carcinoma. A clinicopathologic and immunohistochemical study of 11 cases. Am J Clin Pathol 2000;113:345–350.

20. Soga J, Yakuwa Y, Osaka M. Evaluation of 342 cases of mediastinal/thymic carcinoids collected from literature: a comparative study between typical carcinoids and atypical varieties. Ann Thorac Cardiovasc Surg 1999;5:285–292.

21. Tiffet O, Nicholson AG, Ladas G, Sheppard MN, Goldstraw P. A clinicopathologic study of 12 neuroendocrine tumors arising in the thymus. Chest 2003;124:141–146.

22. Travis WD, Sobin LH. Histological typing of lung and pleural tumours. 3rd edn. In: International histological classification of tumours; no. 1, 1999, Berlin; New York: Springer-Verlag. xii, p. 156.

23. Oliveira AM, Tazelaar HD, Myers JL, Erickson LA, Lloyd RV. Thyroid transcription factor-1 distinguishes metastatic pulmonary from well-differentiated neuroendocrine tumors of other sites. Am J Surg Pathol 2001;25:815–819.

24. Pomplun S, Wotherspoon AC, Shah G, Goldstraw P, Ladas G, Nicholson AG. Immunohistochemical markers in the differentiation of thymic and pulmonary neoplasms. Histopathology 2002;40:152–158.

Radiology

8

Fergus Gleeson and Kirsty Anderson

Introduction

Radiology plays an important role in the investigation of patients with suspected thymic pathology. Imaging may detect incidental disease, confirm suspected disease, stage thymic malignancy, guide biopsy, gauge treatment response and occasionally enable an exact pathological diagnosis, for instance in thymic lipomas. To correctly interpret the appearance on plain chest radiography (CXR), computerised tomographic (CT) scans or magnetic resonance imaging (MRI), it is essential to know the normal appearances of the thymus as it changes through childhood, adolescence and adulthood. This chapter discusses the appearance of the normal thymus, and the imaging appearances of diseases of the thymus.

The Normal Thymus

Recognition of the variety of appearances of the normal thymus on all imaging modalities is necessary to avoid mistaking it for a mediastinal mass and to allow pathology to be identified. On plain radiographs it is usually very prominent at birth, remaining easily visible until the age of two to three years. After this it is inconstantly seen. It causes smooth bilateral superior mediastinal widening on a frontal film, (Fig. 8.1) and lies in the retrosternal space on the lateral film, where it is continuous with the superior cardiac margin (Fig. 8.2). There is sometimes a notch at the junction between the thymic and cardiac silhouettes. It frequently has a variably irregular or "wavy contour" due to indentation by overlying anterior ribs. In approximately 5% of infants, one lobe – most commonly the right – or occasionally both lobes, have a triangular configuration and are more prominent than usual on the frontal film producing a sail sign [1].

The normal thymus is seen on cross sectional imaging such as MRI or CT until patients are in their fourth or fifth decade. It is located in the anterior mediastinum, usually in front of the proximal ascending aorta, pulmonary outflow tract or distal superior vena cava. Its size is dependent on age, but may also appear to vary on respiration, decreasing on inspiration. In a CT study of 154 patients, Baron et al found that the normal thymus was seen in all patients until the age of 39 years; 73% of patients between 30 and 49 years; and only 17% of patients over 49 years. It reached its maximum radiological size between 12 and 19 years [2].

On CT the thymus gland usually has a quadrilateral shape, with convex lateral borders in young children. In patients older than six years, Baron et al found that the majority of thymus glands (62%) had an arrowhead appearance (Fig. 8.3). Visibly distinct right and left lobes showing a variety of shapes (ovoid, elliptical, semilunar or triangular) were found in 32%, and 6% had only one visible lobe. The left lobe was usually larger than the right. In a similar study of 309 patients, Francis et al found that the normal thymus gland never exhibited multilobularity, which can be a useful feature in differentiating normal and abnormal glands [3]. In addition, the normal thymus should conform to the shape of the adjacent great vessels without causing compression or indentation.

As well as a decrease in size, fatty replacement of the thymus with age results in a decrease in CT attenuation values. In patients younger than 19 years, the attenuation is similar to or slightly greater than chest wall muscle, whereas in older patients it approaches that of fat. As the thymus involutes, there may be some residual soft tissue in the mediastinum (Fig. 8.4). In patients over 40 years this usually is in the form of linear or oval soft tissue densities, less than 7 mm in short axis diameter, and should not produce focal alteration in the lateral contour of the mediastinal fat [3].

The thymus is also well seen on MRI. In one small study of 18 patients, the thymus was visible in all patients irrespective of age [4]. In younger patients it has a homogeneous signal intensity, which on T1-weighted images is slightly higher than muscle, and lower than that of mediastinal fat. After puberty, the signal intensity on T1-weighted images increases and the gland may appear less homogeneous due to increased fat content. In older patients the T1 signal can be very similar to that of the mediastinal fat. On T2-weighted images the thymus returns high signal, higher than that of muscle and similar to fat.

Ultrasound can be a useful imaging modality in children. Axial images are obtained via the suprasternal

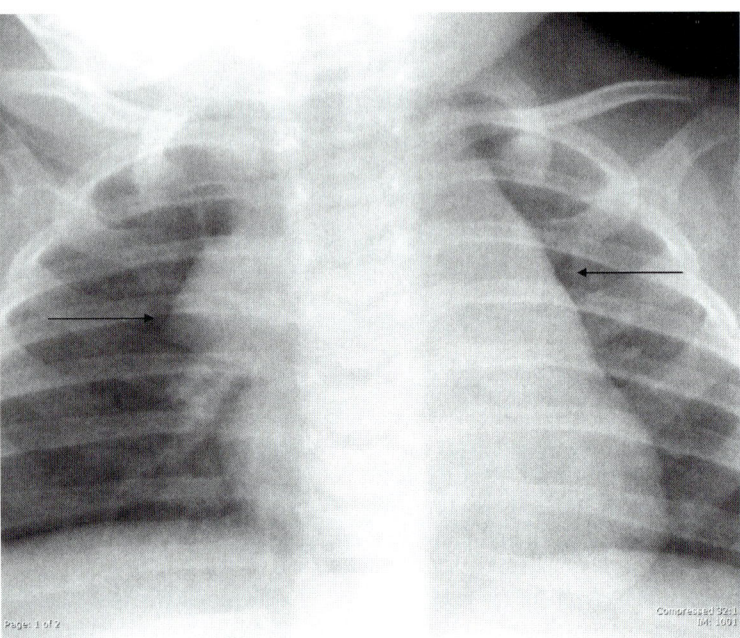

Fig. 8.1 The normal thymus, *arrowed*, seen on CXR, demonstrating widening of the mediastinum. The appearances overall produce the sail sign, and note the normal notch between the right thymic border and the heart beneath the right *arrow*

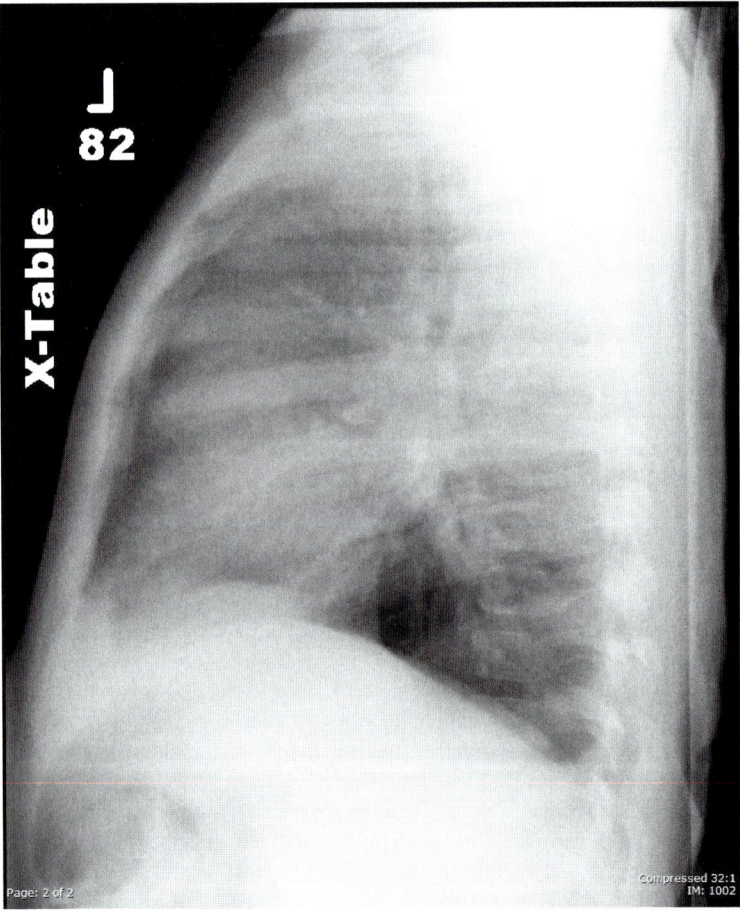

Fig. 8.2 On this lateral CXR, there is infilling of the retrosternal space due to normal thymus

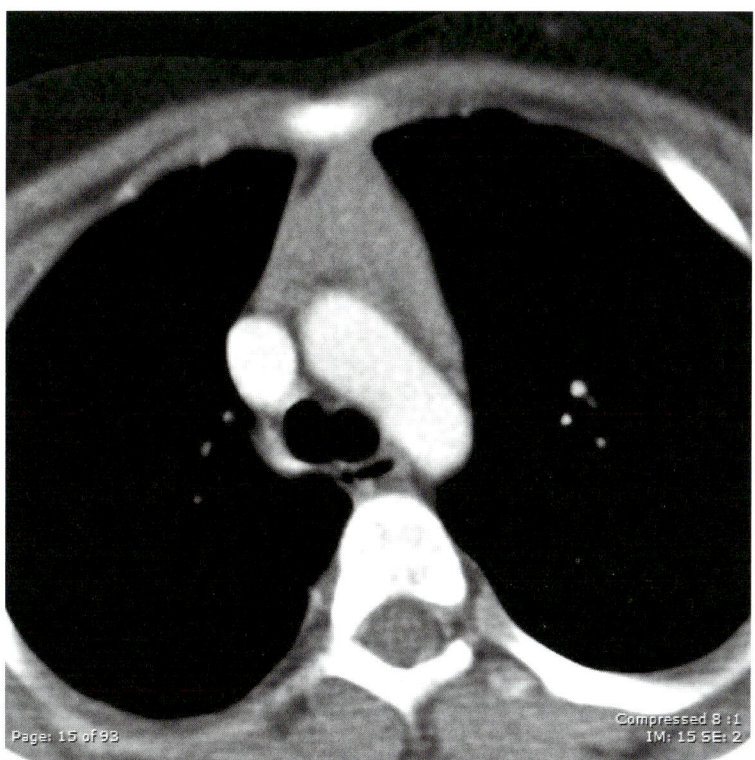

Fig. 8.3 The normal thymus appears as an *arrowhead* within the anterior mediastinum on this contrast enhanced CT

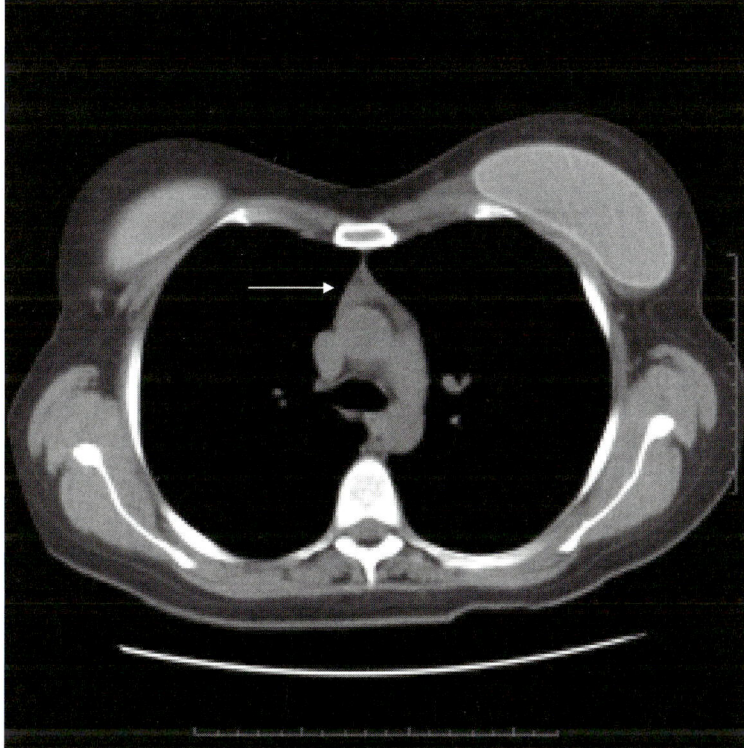

Fig. 8.4 The thymus, seen on this contrast enhanced CT, is part involuted in the anterior mediastinum of this 40-year-old woman

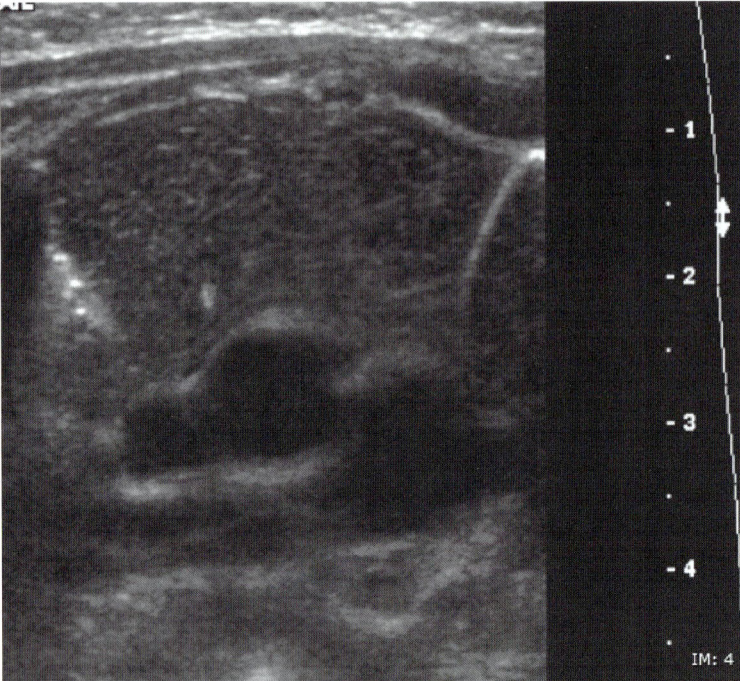

Fig. 8.5 On this ultrasound of the anterior mediastinum in a neonate, the thymus is seen as a homogeneously echogenic mass lying anterior to the great vessels. Note its quadrilateral shape, and the way it is moulded to the shape of the great vessels

notch, and on these images the thymus appears quadrilateral in shape (Fig. 8.5). Longitudinal scans are obtained by scanning intercostally on either side of the sternum. The right lobe tends to have a tear drop appearance, and the left lobe tend to have a triangular or sickle shape [5]. It is of similar echogenicity to liver and spleen, and should be homogeneous. As on other cross sectional imaging, the normal thymus should mould to the shape of adjacent great vessels and should not compress them.

The appearance of the normal thymus with fluorine-18 fluorodeoxyglucose (FDG) PET imaging also varies with age. There is physiological uptake of FDG in the thymus of children and in young adults to a variable degree (Fig. 8.6). There is a correlation between FDG uptake and the CT attenuation value of the thymus, with decreased uptake being seen as the attenuation decreases, owing to fatty replacement. Physiological uptake is not normally seen in patients over 30, although it has been reported in older patients after chemotherapy and radioiodine treatment [6].

Congenital Abnormalities and Normal Variants

Normal variations in thymic location can occur, with ectopic thymic tissue, either separate from or continuous with the normal thymus. It may extend posteriorly,

behind the SVC on the right, or on the left parallel to the aortic arch, into the middle or even posterior mediastinum and may simulate a mediastinal mass. Ectopic thymic tissue can also occur as a result of migrational defects during thymic embryogenesis. It may be found anywhere along a line from the angle of the mandible to the sternal notch, and in the anterior mediastinum down to the level of the diaphragm, although it is most commonly reported in the neck, where it can occasionally be seen compressing the airways. It can be mistaken for lymph node or tumour. Despite its ectopic position, it usually has the same characteristics as a normal thymus on all imaging modalities relative to the patient's age, although occasionally it is seen as a cystic mass.

The thymus may be entirely absent, as in patients with DiGeorge syndrome. On plain radiographs this may be suggested by a narrow superior mediastinum, but CT or MRI is required to distinguish complete absence from thymic hypoplasia or stress atrophy.

Thymic Pathology

Thymic Hyperplasia

Thymic hyperplasia is rarely visible on plain film. On CT and MRI the gland is diffusely enlarged, especially in its transverse diameter, although often the size will still lie

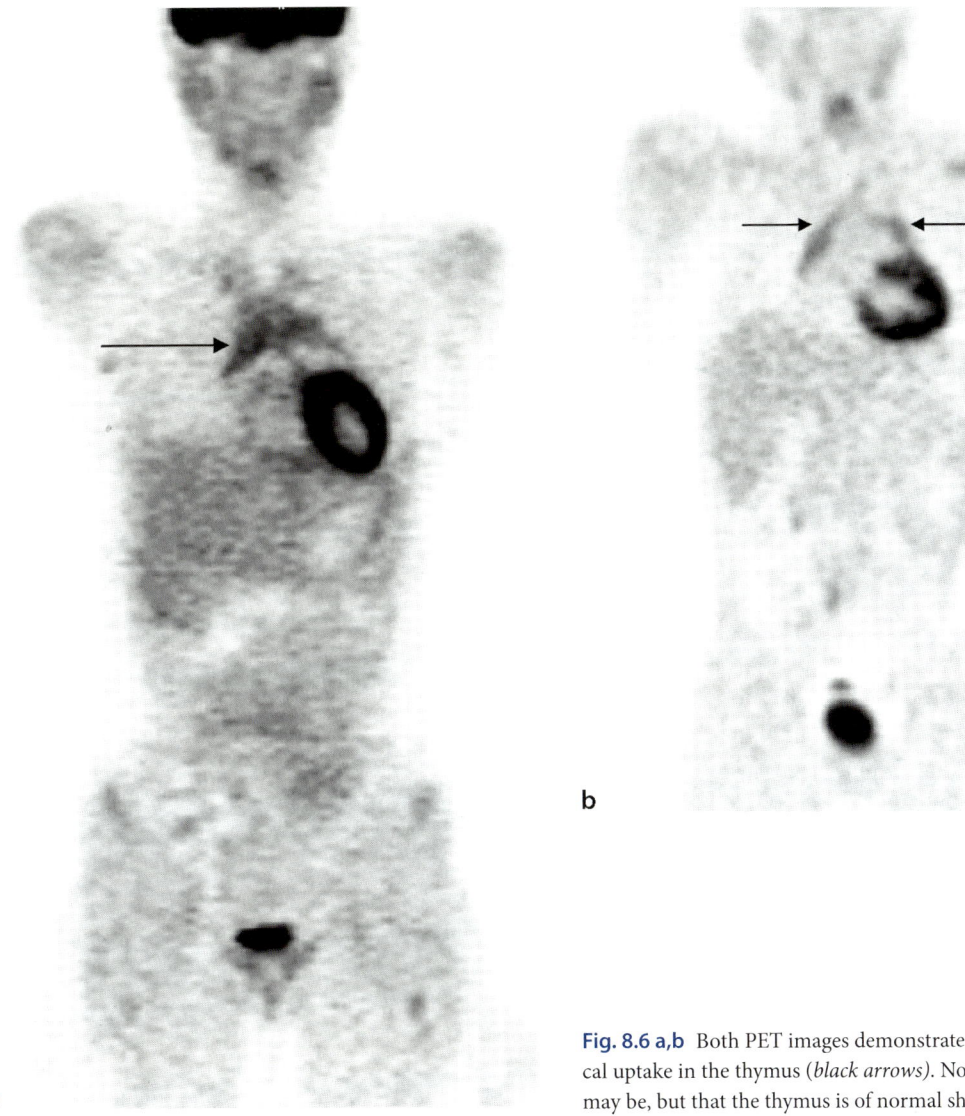

a

b

Fig. 8.6 a,b Both PET images demonstrate normal physiological uptake in the thymus (*black arrows*). Note how variable this may be, but that the thymus is of normal shape in both patients

within the normal range and the diagnosis will be made post resection at histopathology. Normal shape and attenuation or signal intensity are usually preserved. Cases have been reported, however, of hyperplasia causing focal masses in patients with myasthenia [7]. Thymic hyperplasia may occur due to rebound hypertrophy following a period of stress such as post-chemotherapy, but again, other than an increase in size, imaging characteristics should be the same as for normal thymus. Differentiation from tumour infiltration and potential disease relapse, for instance in patients with lymphoma, is frequently not possible using CT or MRI characterisation alone. Symmetrical enlargement and preservation of normal signal on MRI are suggestive of rebound, and review of the other areas of the scan for exclusion of disease relapse at other sites and clinical correlation is mandatory.

Thymoma

On the plain CXR a thymoma, if large, will be seen as a soft tissue mass in the anterior mediastinum (Fig. 8.7). They are often spherical and may have smooth or lobulated margins. Smaller tumours will not be seen on plain film, although up to 75% of thymomas have been reported as visible on CXR [8]. Most commonly, they are seen in the anterior and superior mediastinum, but may be seen adjacent to the cardiac border or in the cardiophrenic angles, and rarely in the neck or middle and posterior mediastinum.

CT is the most commonly used imaging modality for the detection and staging of thymomas. Thymomas are usually seen as homogeneous soft tissue masses in the anterior mediastinum. They most often have a smooth or

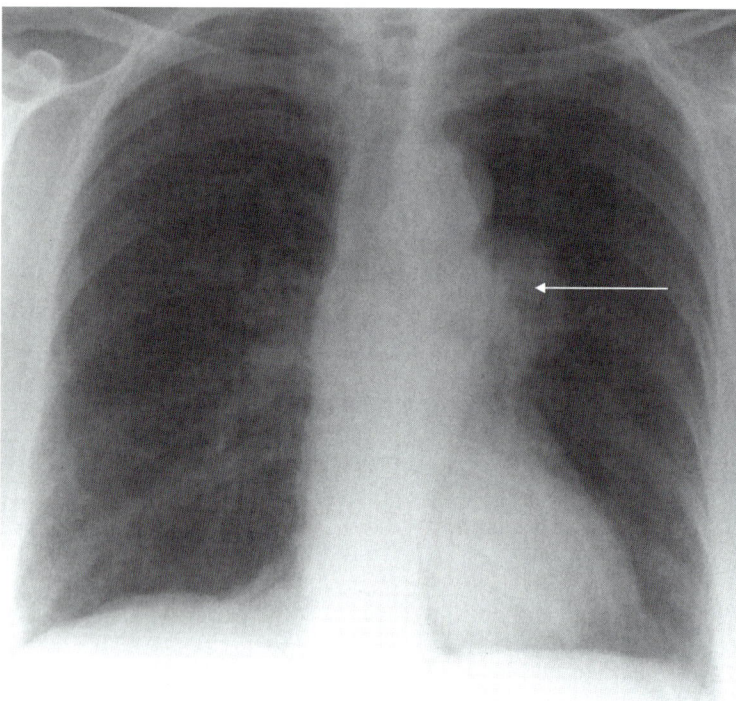

Fig. 8.7 a An anterior mediastinal mass is seen (*arrow*) on this PA CXR. **b** A contrast enhanced CT of the same patient demonstrates the mass is a thymoma. It is seen to enhance (*white arrow*) and contains areas of calcification (*black arrow*)

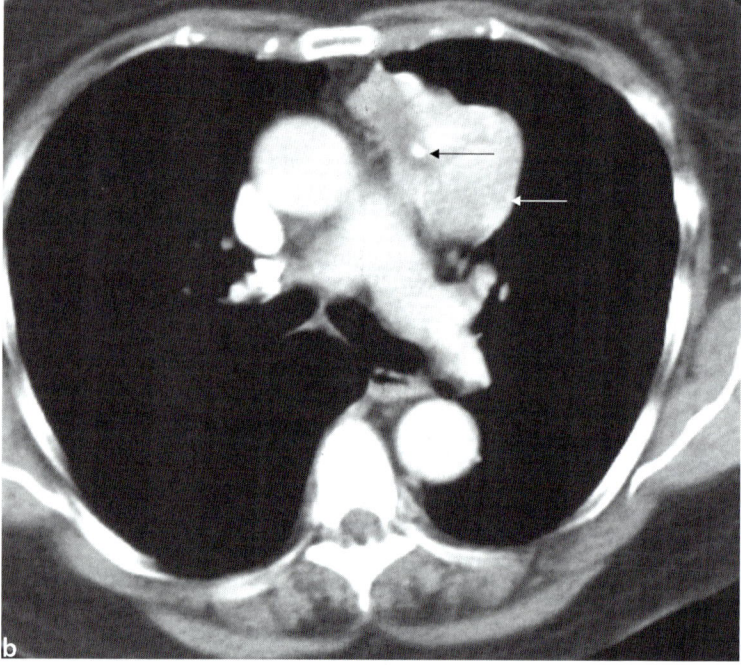

lobulated contour and are round or oval (Fig. 8.8). They may displace the heart and great vessels. Calcification is present in 5–25% [9], and is often thin, linear and peripheral. This may be seen on plain film, but CT is more sensitive. There may be focal areas of decreased attenuation due to cystic change, necrosis or haemorrhage. Nodules may arise from the inner walls of cysts within a thymoma.

They enhance uniformly post intravenous contrast (although cystic or necrotic areas will not enhance).

Recognising focal swellings or masses within the thymus becomes easier as the thymus atrophies with age. Tumours as small as 1.5 cm can be identified in patients older than 40 years. In younger patients the normal gland may be larger, making small thymomas harder to detect

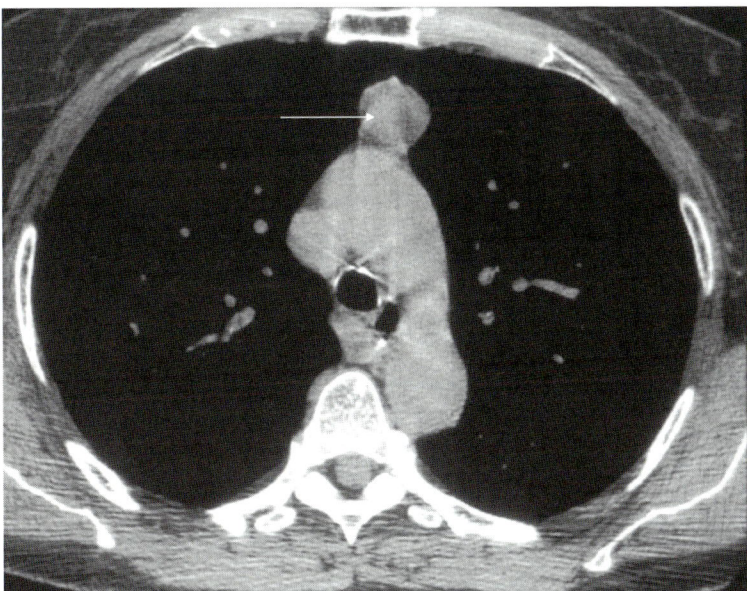

Fig. 8.8 A contrast enhanced CT demonstrates a homogeneously enhancing, smooth bordered, non-invasive, encapsulated thymoma (*white arrow*) in the anterior mediastinum

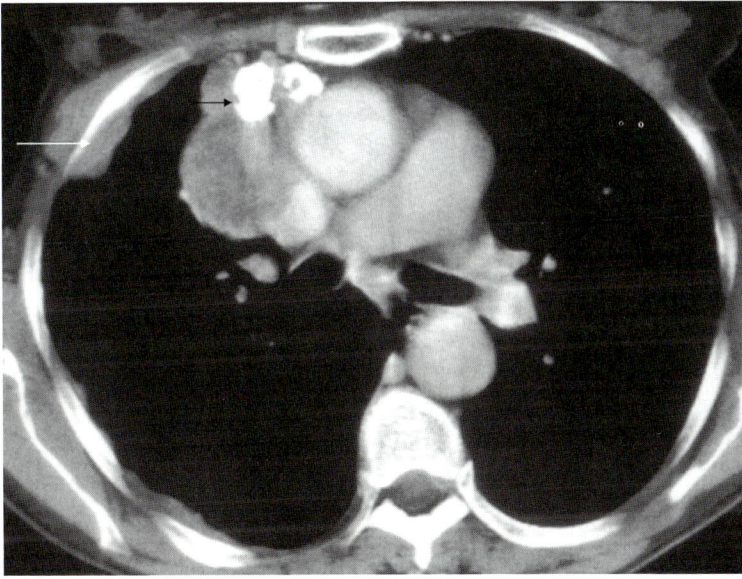

Fig. 8.9 A contrast enhanced CT demonstrating an invasive thymoma, with areas of dense calcification (*black arrow*) and transpleural spread (*white arrow*)

unless they give rise to asymmetric focal swelling. Fortunately, thymoma is rare in children, when detection becomes even harder.

CT can help to identify invasive disease, although it is not reliable in this respect. If the tumour is confined to the thymus, the adjacent mediastinal fat planes will be preserved – although preservation of fat planes does not exclude capsular involvement. Complete obliteration of surrounding fat planes is suggestive of mediastinal invasion, but partial obliteration can occur with local inflammatory change [10].

CT also detects transpleural spread, both locally and as drop metastases distant from the primary lesion (Fig. 8.9). Pleural disease can be so extensive as to mimic mesothelioma. Although extra-thoracic metastases are rare, transdiaphragmatic spread of pleural tumour into the retroperitoneum has been described. The entire thorax and upper abdomen, therefore, should be imaged in a patient with suspected invasive disease.

MRI can provide further useful information, particularly with respect to the local extent of the thymoma and invasiveness. Thymoma has a similar signal intensity to muscle on T1-weighted images, and on T2-weighted images is slightly heterogeneous with signal intensity similar to fat (Fig. 8.10) [11]. MRI can be useful in differentiating hyperplasia from thymoma by demonstrating the normal shape and signal of the gland in the former. It can help to differentiate a thymic mass from other

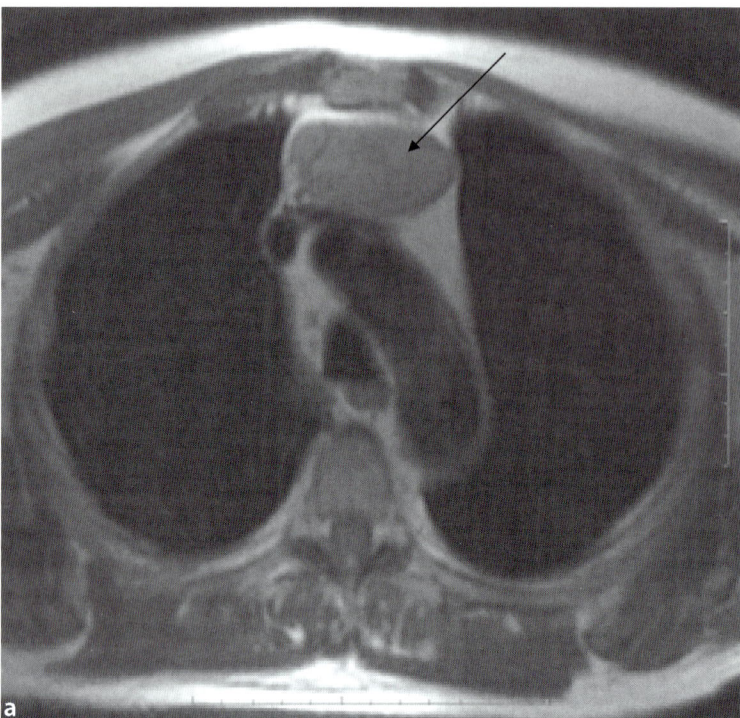

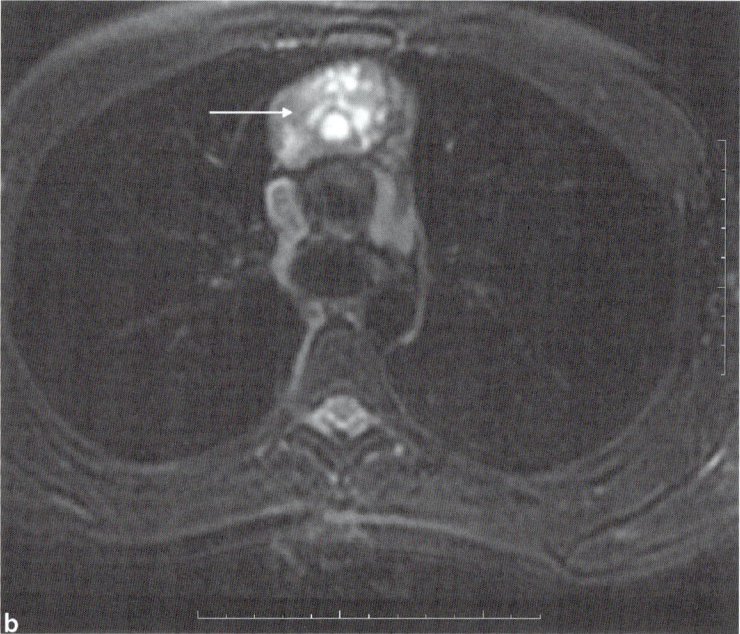

Fig. 8.10 a A T1-weighted MRI sequence, demonstrating a smooth bordered thymoma (*black arrow*) seen within the fat of the anterior mediastinum. **b** A fat saturated T2-weighted MRI sequence, demonstrating the thymoma (*white arrow*). Note the heterogeneous and increased signal intensity, compared to other structures

mediastinal masses by demonstrating the median raphe separating the two lobes, thereby confirming that the lesion is thymic. Invasive thymomas characteristically are less well defined and have more heterogeneous signal. On T2-weighted images, internal septation and loculation may be seen with intralocular variation in signal intensity (Fig. 8.11) [12]. In invasive disease, it is more reliable than CT in assessing invasion of local structures

such as the pericardium and great vessels and, therefore, helps to determine operability. It has also been shown to be better than CT in detecting tumour recurrence after surgery [13].

Dynamic MR imaging has been used to help distinguish thymomas from other mediastinal tumours. By obtaining sequential images at 30-second intervals after intravenous gadolinium administration, time intensity

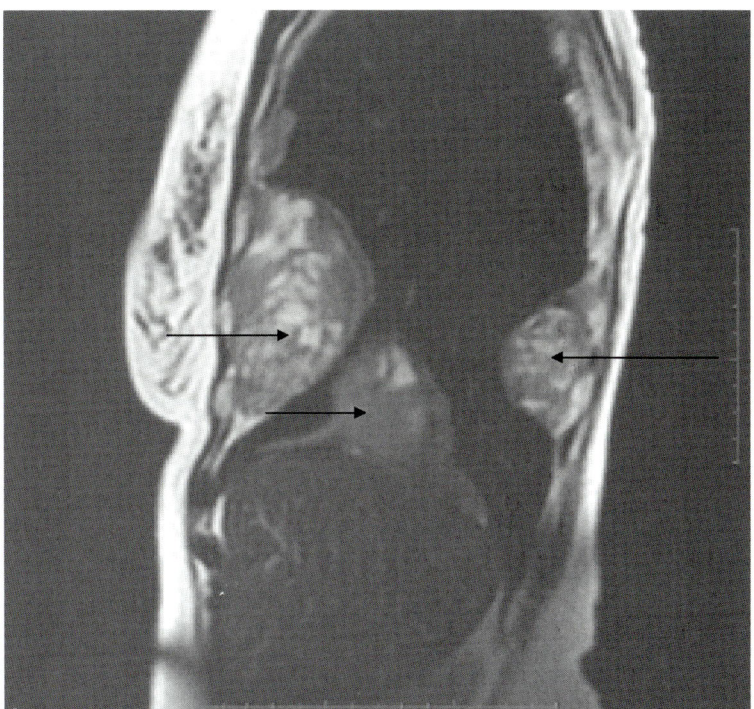

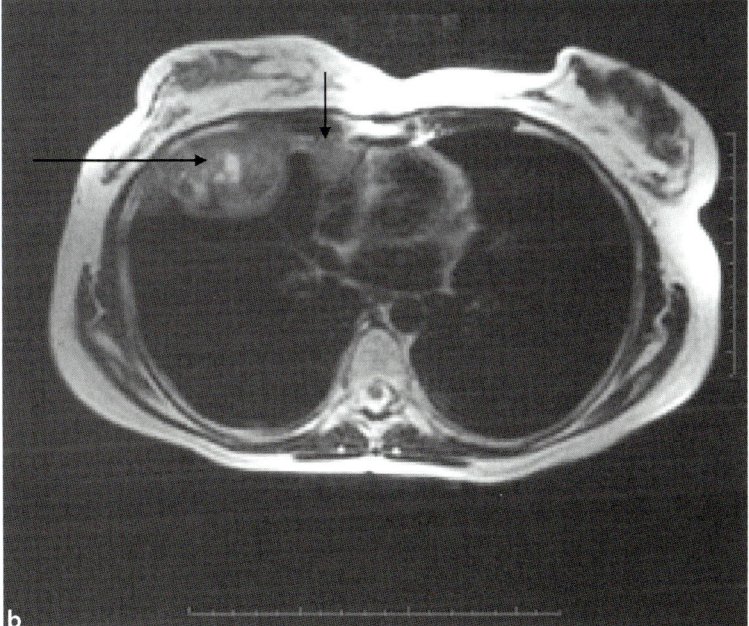

Fig. 8.11 a, b Metastatic thymoma, seen as heterogeneous signal intensity pleural metastases (*arrow*) on these T2-weighted axial and coronal MRI sequences

curves (TIC) can be generated. Thymoma tends to reach a peak in TIC relatively early (less than 2.5 min.), with other tumours such as thymic carcinoma, lymphoma, germ cell tumour and carcinoid having later peaks [14].

Scintigraphy using thallium 201 has been used to evaluate thymic lesions in patients with myasthenia. It can help differentiate normal thymus, thymic hyperplasia and thymoma. Increased thallium uptake is detected on both early and delayed images in thymoma, whereas in thymic hyperplasia more intense uptake is seen on the delayed images than the early images. This may be more sensitive in the detection of thymic hyperplasia than CT [15].

Indium 111 labelled octreotide has also been used in the detection of thymoma and other thymic tumours. It is avidly concentrated in thymic tumours such as thymoma, thymic carcinoma and thymic carcinoid, but not in thymic hyperplasia or the normal thymus [16].

Thymic Carcinoma

Thymic carcinomas are less common than thymomas. They have often invaded adjacent structures at the time of diagnosis. Radiological appearances are similar to those of invasive thymoma, with an anterior mediastinal mass which may have areas of calcification, necrosis, haemorrhage and cystic change. Some studies report that they have a relatively low signal on both T1- and T2-weighted MR images compared with thymomas [17]. As with invasive thymoma they may have heterogeneous signal on MR. It has also been reported that, on average, carcinomas tend to be larger than thymomas and that invasion of the great vessels, lymph node enlargement, haematogenous metastases and phrenic nerve palsy are more indicative of carcinoma [18].

Thymic Carcinoid

Radiographic features of thymic carcinoids are non-specific. On plain radiographs and CT, they appear as lobulated anterior mediastinal masses, occasionally with calcification. They may be well differentiated or aggressive, and the latter may invade adjacent structures such as pleura, pericardium, diaphragm and mediastinum. They are not distinguishable from thymoma on CT. On MRI they are hypointense on T1-weighted images, and inhomogeneously hyperintense on T2 [19].

Cushing's syndrome is seen in 33–40% of patients with thymic carcinoids [20]. Those tumours associated with Cushing's syndrome tend to be smaller at presentation and are less likely to be visible on plain radiographs. They may also be too small to detect on cross sectional imaging. In patients with Cushing's syndrome and normal MRI and CT, scintigraphy using Indium 111 labelled octreotide may localise the tumour, although this is not specific for carcinoid. The hypercortisolaemia found in Cushing's syndrome does not significantly affect the appearance of the thymus in patients without thymic carcinoids. In these patients the size of the thymus varies with age in the same way as in the normal population [21].

Thymic carcinoid commonly metastasises to regional lymph nodes, skin, adrenals and bones. As with carcinoids arising in other sites, the bone metastases are usually osteoblastic and so appear sclerotic on plain films.

Lymphoma

The thymus may be a site of involvement of lymphoma and leukaemia (Fig. 8.12) particularly the nodular sclerosing type of Hodgkin's disease, where it is involved in 40–50% of cases. It is usually part of generalised disease, although isolated involvement can occur. Radiographic features are not specific, and it is not distinguishable from other solid thymic tumours. There may be areas of

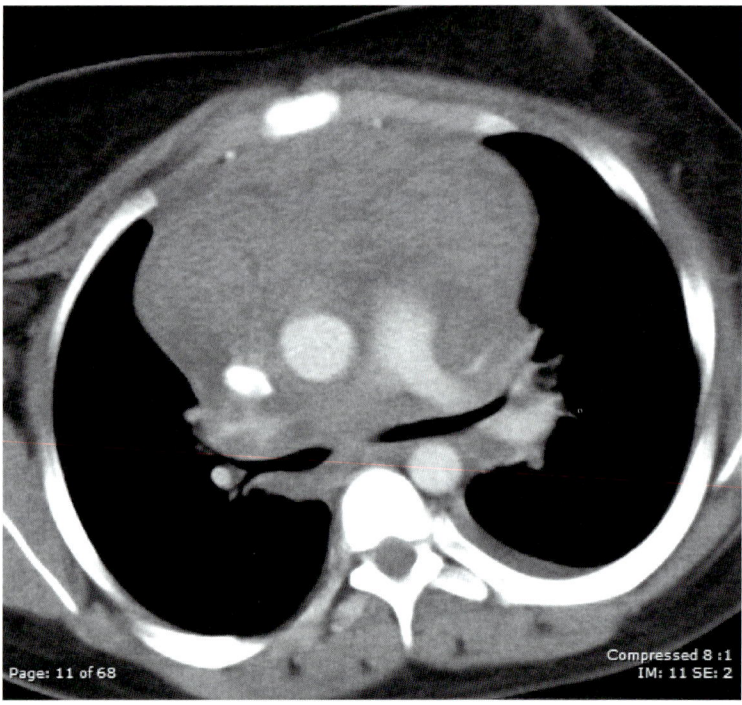

Fig. 8.12 On this contrast enhanced CT scan, there is a very large anterior mediastinal mass. Note the slight heterogeneous enhancement in keeping with cystic degeneration. Biopsy confirmed non-Hodgkins lymphoma

cystic degeneration. The presence of mediastinal or hilar lymphadenopathy should suggest the diagnosis.

On MRI the thymus often becomes low signal on both T1- and T2-weighted images post treatment for lymphoma due to fibrosis. Persistent high signal on T2-weighting, however, may occur due to post treatment change, inflammation or haemorrhage, in addition to recurrent lymphoma [22]. In younger patients it can be difficult to distinguish recurrent lymphoma from rebound thymic hyperplasia after treatment. Hyperplasia and malignant infiltration may show similar CT attenuation and MR signal intensity. The hyperplastic gland should retain a normal non-lobulated outline and conform to the shape of adjacent structures. Enlargement should be symmetrical in hyperplasia, but is usually asymmetrical with tumour involvement. If there is marked non-homogeneity of signal on MR imaging, then this suggests malignant disease rather than hyperplasia.

Thymolipoma/Liposarcoma

Thymolipomas are rare thymic tumours consisting of fat and interspersed residual thymic tissue. They can be very large and may slump inferiorly from the anterior mediastinum to the diaphragm. They mould themselves to mediastinal structures and diaphragm, but do not compress or invade mediastinal structures. On plain radiographs they may mimic cardiomegaly, diaphragmatic elevation or lobar collapse. On CT they are predominantly of fat density and have fibrous strands and areas of normal thymic tissue within them. On MRI they are of high signal on both T1- and T2-weighted sequences, and may contain lower signal strands. A connection between the thymus and the tumour should be seen on both CT and MRI.

Thymoliposarcoma is a rare tumour of adulthood. There is little literature regarding its radiological appearance, but in a single case report it was predominantly of soft tissue density on CT, containing only small areas of fat attenuation [23].

Thymic Cyst

Thymic cysts may be congenital or acquired secondary to surgery or treated Hodgkin's disease. They may be unilocular or multilocular, and have been reported up to 18 cm in size. On plain film they appear similar to other thymic masses. Calcification in the wall has been reported. On CT the cyst contents is usually of fluid attenuation, although if the contents is proteinaceous or haemorrhagic then attenuation values will be higher and it may appear solid. On MRI they are very high signal on T2-weighted images and usually low signal on T1 weighting. The contents may have higher T1 signal if there is haemorrhage or high protein content. Cyst contents should not enhance post intravenous contrast on CT or MRI.

Germ Cell Tumours

Mediastinal germ cell tumours are almost always found in the anterior mediastinum in the region of the thymus. On cross sectional imaging, non-seminomatous germ

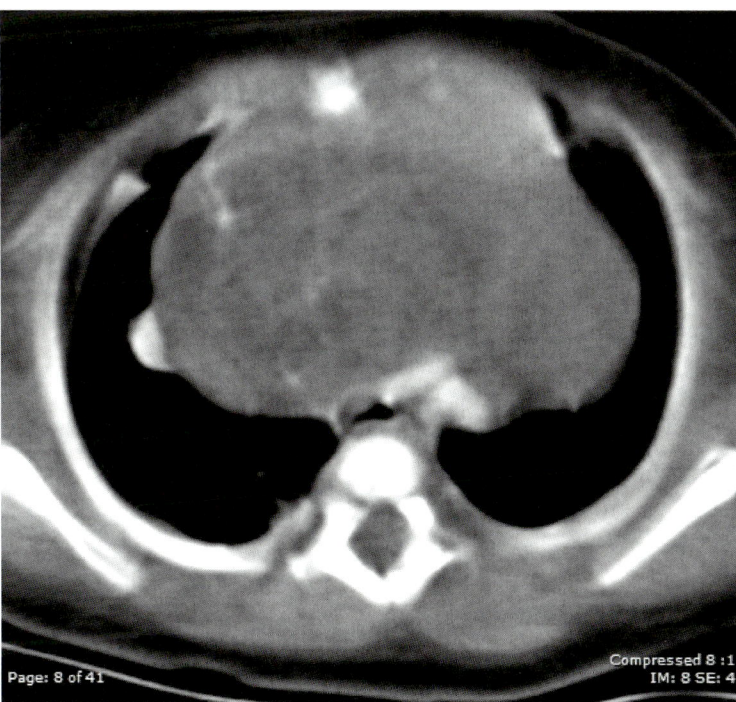

Fig. 8.13 A contrast enhanced CT, demonstrating a massive anterior mediastinal mass, with areas of low attenuation, heterogeneous enhancement and calcification. This was a germ cell tumour on biopsy

cell tumours are non-homogeneous, containing a variable mixture of fat, soft tissue, calcification and haemorrhagic components (Fig. 8.13). Seminomas are usually homogeneous and, therefore, difficult to differentiate from other tumours such as thymoma.

Miscellaneous

Other conditions that may affect the thymus include lymphangioma, haemangioma, metastases and inflammatory processes. Lyphangioma or haemangioma may be suggested on CT and MRI, with both showing abnormal vessels in the thymus. Inflammatory processes such as TB and Langerhan's cell histiocytosis (LCH) produce thymic enlargement. Thymic LCH is usually associated with pulmonary histiocytosis. Fine calcification and cavitation have been reported on CT.

References

1. Day DL, Gedgaudas E. The thymus. Radiol Clin North Am 1984; 22:519.
2. Baron RL, Lee JKT, Sagel SS, et al. Computed tomography of the normal thymus. Radiology 1982; 142:121–125.
3. Francis IR, Glazer GM, Bookstein FL, et al. The thymus: re-examination of age-related changes in size and shape. AJR 1985; 145:249–254.
4. de Geer G, Webb R, Gamsu G. Normal thymus: assessment with MR and CT. Radiology 1986; 158:313–317.
5. Adam EJ, Ignotus PI. Sonography of the thymus in healthy children: frequency of visualization, size, and appearance. AJR 1993; 161:153–155.
6. Nakahara T, Fujii H, Ide M, et al. FDG uptake in the morphologically normal thymus: comparison of FDG positron emission tomography and CT. BJR 2001; 74:821–824.
7. Nicolaou S, Muller NL, Li DKB, et al. Thymus in myasthenia gravis: comparison of CT and pathological findings and clinical outcome after thymectomy. Radiology 1996; 201:471–474.
8. Morgenthaler TI, Brown LR, Colby TV, et al. Thymoma. Mayo Clin Proc 1993; 68:1110–1123.
9. Dahnert W. Radiology review manual. 4th ed. Lippincott, Williams and Wilkins, 2000, Philadelphia, pp 442–443.
10. Chen J, Weisbroad GL, Herman SJ, et al. Computed tomography and pathological correlations of thymic lesions. J Thorac Imag 1988; 3:61–65.
11. Batra P, Herrmann C, Mulder D. Mediastinal imaging in myasthenia gravis: correlation of chest radiography, CT, MR and surgical findings. AJR 1987; 148:515–519.
12. Kono M. MRI diagnosis of thymic tumours and differential diagnosis. Thoracicrad.org
13. Pirronti T, Rinaldi P, Batocchi AP, et al. Thymic lesions and myasthenia gravis. Diagnosis based on mediastinal imaging and pathological findings. Acta Radiol 2002; 43:380–384.
14. Sakai S, Murayama S, Soeda H, et al. Differential diagnosis between thymoma and non-thymoma by dynamic MR imaging. Acta Radiol 2002; 43:262–268.
15. Higuchi T, Taki J, Kinuya S, et al. Thymic lesions in patients with myasthenia gravis: Characterization with thallium 201 scintigraphy. Radiology 2001; 221:201–206.
16. Lastoria S, Vergara E, Palmiera G, et al. In vivo detection of malignant thymic masses by indium-111-DTPA-D-Phe1-octreotide scintigraphy. J Nucl Med 1998; 39:634–639.
17. Kushihashi T, Fujisawa H, Munechika H. Magnetic resonance imaging of thymic epithelial tumors. Crit Rev Diagn Imaging 1996;37:191–259
18. Jung K, Soo Lee K, Han J, et al. Malignant thymic epithelial tumors: CT–pathologic correlation. AJR 2001; 176:433–439.
19. Ferrozzi F, Ganzetti A, Mugnoli E et al. Thymic carcinoid: CT and MR findings. Radiol Med (Torino) 1997;94:652–656.
20. Rosado de Christenson ML, Abbott GF, Kirejczyk WM, et al. Thoracic carcinoids: radiologic-pathologic correlation. Radiographics 1999; 19:707–736.
21. Hanson JA, Sohaib SA, Newell-Price J et al. Computed tomography appearance of the thymus and anterior mediastinum in active Cushing's syndrome. J Clin Endocrinol and Metab 1999; 84:602–605.
22. Molina PL, Siegel MJ, Glazer HS. Thymic masses on MR imaging. AJR 1990; 155:495–500.
23. Howling SJ, Flint JDA, Muller NL. Thymoliposarcoma: CT and pathologic findings. Clin Radiol 1999; 54:341.

Thymectomy

9

Kyriakos Anastasiadis and Chandi Ratnatunga

Introduction

Thymectomy for MG was first reported by Sauerbruch in 1913 [1]. It became accepted as a therapeutic option for myasthenia gravis after Blalock et al. first performed this procedure in 1936 and described its technique in 1939 [2]. Blalock, who pioneered thymectomy in the management of MG, reported the results of his first six MG patients, who improved after surgical removal of thymus in 1941 [3], and advocated the extension of thymectomy to the treatment of non-thymomatous patients with MG [4]. Keynes in London and Eaton et al. from the Mayo Clinic followed by reporting similarly good results from thymectomy in myasthenic patients [5, 6].

The fact that three-quarters of MG patients have abnormalities of the thymus (commonly hyperplasia of the gland) [7] and one-tenth of patients have thymoma, established the surgical removal of the gland as a popular method in the management of the disease. The introduction of immunosuppressive therapy in conjunction with thymectomy decreased the mortality of the disease from 26% to <5% [8, 9]. A spontaneous remission rate for MG in untreated patients of only 20% [10, 11], compared to reports of complete remission in up to 50% and of clinical improvement as high as 97% after thymectomy, further consolidated the position of surgery as a therapeutic modality for MG.

This surgical success led trans-sternal thymectomy to become the "standard" approach. With time, other surgical approaches were introduced; Crile in 1966 introduced the trans-cervical approach [12] and was soon followed by Kirschner et al. [13]. Masaoka et al. in 1975 demonstrated that ectopic thymic tissue could be found in the mediastinal fat of the majority of patients [14]. Following Masoaka's observations Jaretzki and Wolff studied and then described what is now accepted as the normal surgical anatomy of the thymus, defining the findings as "variation" and not "ectopic" (Fig. 9.13). Based on these anatomical findings the "total", later revised to "maximal", thymectomy was developed by Jaretzki [15, 16]. The spectrum of approaches in the modern era of thymectomy now stretches from minimally invasive techniques, such as transcervical and endoscopic approaches, to the

"classical" trans-sternal approach with modifications (partial sternotomy), to maximal thymectomy.

The computer-assisted matched study of Buckingham et al. [17] found that 33% of patients who underwent thymectomy for MG experienced complete remission, compared to only 8% of those treated medically. The 5- and 10-year survival in myasthenic patients, furthermore, was better with surgery than with medical treatment alone (Fig. 9.1). In a recent meta-analysis of long-term results of thymectomy, 90% of MG patients who underwent surgery improved, 80% became asymptomatic and 50% achieved complete remission [18]. These studies merely established the case for surgery to treat MG. Surgery also became a recognised treatment strategy in the management of thymic enlargement of neoplastic or non-neoplastic origin.

When the decision to recommend surgery is made, a thorough pre-operative evaluation and preparation of the patient on a multidisciplinary basis (surgeon, neurologist, radiologist and anaesthetist) is essential (see also chapters 5, 8, 10). Accurate imaging (usually CT or MRI scanning) is of utmost importance to the surgeon, particularly in identifying thymomas and the extent of their invasion locally. This provides the necessary information for designing the surgical strategy. Actual thymic size is of less importance than the relationship of the gland and tumour to adjacent structures, which could predict the possibility of resection and the need for support facilities at the time of surgery, such as cardiopulmonary bypass, cell savers and cardiothoracic anaesthesia. The appropriate preparation of myasthenic patients for thymectomy and their management after surgery needs careful neurological, anaesthetic and intensivist input, and are dealt with in chapters 5, 8, 10 of this book.

Indications for Thymectomy

Thymectomy is the gold standard treatment in all patients with thymic tumours, but its position is more controversial in non-thymomatous MG patients. The criteria for thymectomy are not clear despite the general acceptance that thymectomy is a valuable tool in the management

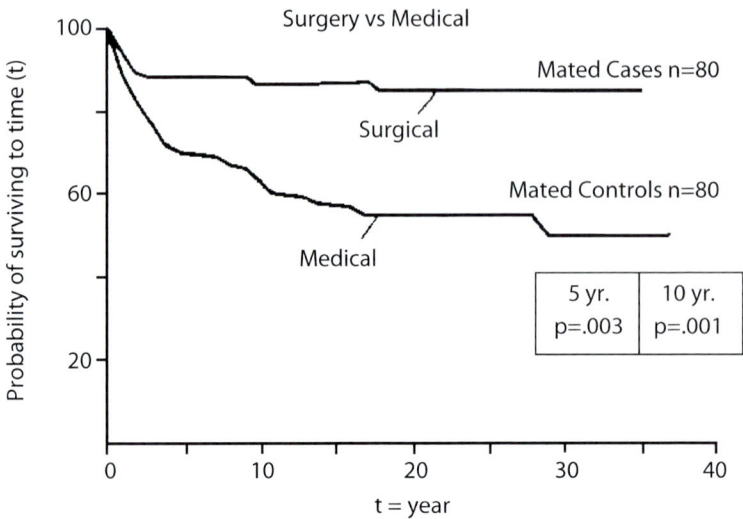

Fig. 9.1 Comparison of survival between MG patients treated surgically and medically [17] (Used with permission)

of MG, particularly in those refractory to conservative management [19–21]. Lanska, who surveyed the referral practice of neurologists for thymectomy, found that >50% advocated the procedure for between one-third and two-thirds of their patients, and that 33% advocated the procedure for more than two-thirds of their patients, but that <10% advocated the procedure for less than one-third of their patients. Their referral criteria were: patients with thymoma, generalised MG unresponsive to medical management and ocular disease refractory to medical management [23].

There is no true consensus among the medical profession, however, about indications for thymectomy in MG. The relevance of thymectomy at one extreme end of the disease spectrum is clearer: most patients with late-severe generalised disease have poor response to thymectomy, as well as a high morbidity and mortality rate, and therefore are poor surgical candidates [9]. At the other end of the spectrum, in those patients with purely ocular symptoms, although good control can be achieved with drugs, there are reports that thymectomy produces good results (e.g. up to 70% improvement rate [24]). The indication for thymectomy is more controversial here, but conventional wisdom suggests that thymectomy is indicated in disabled patients in the early stages of the disease [25] or in patients with resistant disease refractory to conservative therapy [20]. There is an even greater lack of consensus in the middle of the disease spectrum. Papatestas et al. have proposed early surgical intervention in all MG patients on the basis of good results and because thymectomy reduces the risk of development of extrathymic neoplasms in MG [8]. In line with this, there is a trend towards early surgery in many centres, as evidence does exist that surgical intervention favours outcome [26]. In reality, opinions on the indications for thymectomy in MG patients will reflect the views of the specialities: physicians in general favour medical man-

agement, using surgery as a final resort; surgeons favour early surgery. The authors' opinion is that surgery is indicated in patients with disease refractory to medical management whatever the disease severity, and that early surgical intervention carries benefit. They also feel that surgery should not be denied to patients with very severe disease, although they recognise that they are higher risk and that their chance of remission is poorer, as these individuals have exhausted all other therapeutic options.

The role of age is also controversial. With the bimodal age distribution of MG (with peaks at the second and the seventh decade) the second peak of patients would be excluded if the previously held view that 40 to 50 years of age cut-off for thymectomy is followed. This is increasingly challenged, and thymectomy is now recommended as a safe and effective treatment for elderly patients with MG [27, 28].

Thymectomy Techniques

Trans-sternal Thymectomy

The patient is prepared as discussed in Chapter 10. This approach commences with midline sternotomy, full or partial, which gives excellent exposure to the thymus. The approach also gives the surgeon the option of extension into the neck for exploration of "aberrant" thymic tissue to permit complete resection. Many different skin incisions (usually for cosmetic reasons) have been employed: mid-line, bilateral submammary, "champagne glass", minimal (mini) median, T-incision, etc. [29, 30]. At Oxford, the preferred skin incision is a full midline to obtain good and easy access (Fig. 9.2). Others in contrast are strong advocates of partial sternotomy, because it is less invasive [31].

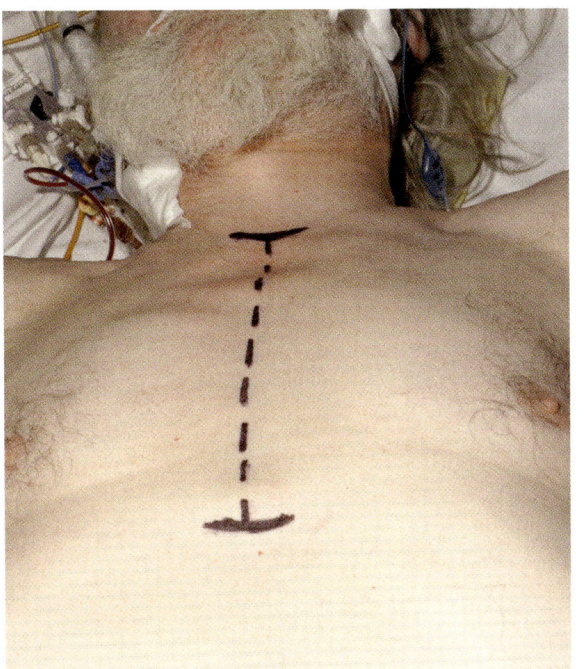

Fig. 9.2 The surface marking for a midline sternotomy incision for trans-sternal thymectomy

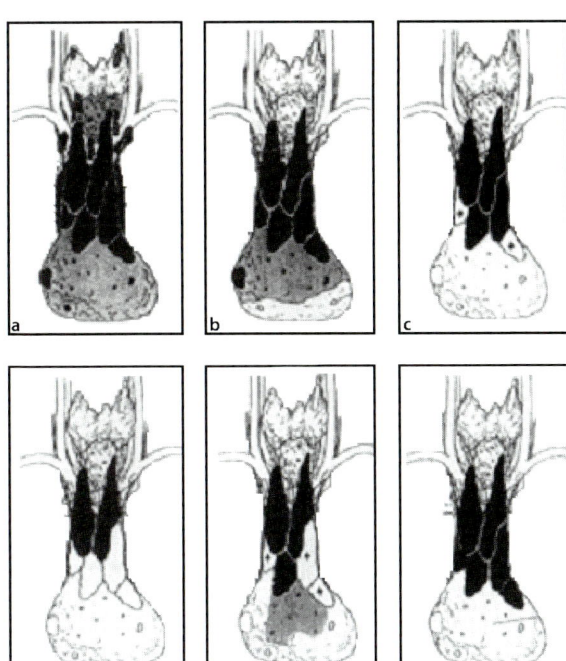

Fig. 9.3 Estimated extent of various thymectomy techniques (**a**: maximal, **b**: extended sternal, **c**: standard sternal, **d**: basic cervical, **e**: extended cervical, **f**: VATS). *Black* = thymus, *gray* = fat that may contain islands of thymus and microscopic thymus, * = thymic lobes or thymofatty tissue that may or may not be removed [55] (Used with permission)

The extent of the thymic resection is described as standard, extended or maximal. By definition these techniques describe the proposed extent of resection of all thymic tissue within the mediastinum and neck. In Fig. 9.3 Jaretzki's estimated extent of resection of thymic tissue by the various transsternal and cervical approaches can be seen [55].

Standard thymectomy consists solely of resection of the gland, while in extended thymectomy all anterior mediastinal fat tissue is removed, along with the thymus. Masaoka et al. [32] demonstrated that an extended thymectomy is superior to standard thymectomy with regard to clinical outcome, and that thymic remnants outside the thymus also play an important role in MG (see also Maximal Thymectomy section, below).

Standard trans-sternal thymectomy continues after sternal haemostasis is achieved [26] with the mobilisation of the thymus from the pericardium posteriorly, and from the mediastinal pleura laterally. This mobilisation commences with the lower poles of the thymic lobes, where it is easiest. The pericardium is not breached unless there is pericardial involvement or invasion. The mobilisation of the thymic tissue from the pleura can be aided by controlled hand ventilation by the anaesthetist. Care should be given to identifying and preserving the phrenic nerves laterally; these ascend towards

the mid-part of the gland and are intimately related to the thymus here, as they pass from the chest into the neck at the level of the thoracic inlet. Preservation of the phrenic nerves in myasthenics is critical to avoid severe post-operative respiratory compromise. The dissection continues, mobilising the thymus together with the extra-pleural fat. In most cases dissection can be performed without damage to the pleura, but breaching the pleural lining is not in itself a matter of great concern. If this occurs, however, it must be recognised to avoid a pneumothorax. As mobilisation continues in a cephalic direction, the arterial supply, which enters the gland laterally, usually in the form of two branches to each lobe, is encountered and divided between surgical clips. Centrally, the sharp dissection is carried usually superficial to the innominate vein. In the unusual case, however, the thymus extends in a cephalic direction posterior or deep to the vein.

The venous drainage of the gland, usually two or three small veins, is identified and divided between surgical clips. The sharp dissection leaves the innominate vein bare. The upper pole (cervical extensions) of the lobes are finally mobilised by retraction of the strap muscles. These poles may extend surprisingly high into the neck, and care must be taken to ensure their complete removal (Fig. 9.4). The thymus is finally freed by

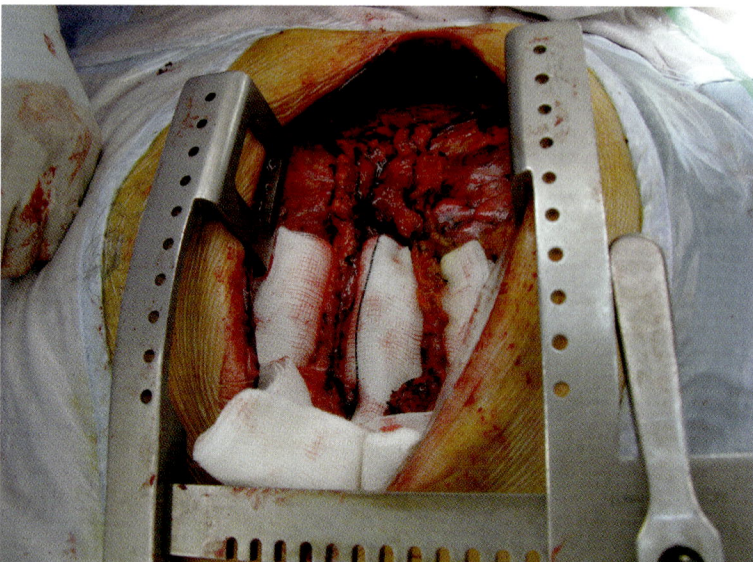

Fig. 9.4 The mobilised and dissected upper poles of the thymus on a surgical swab (white material)

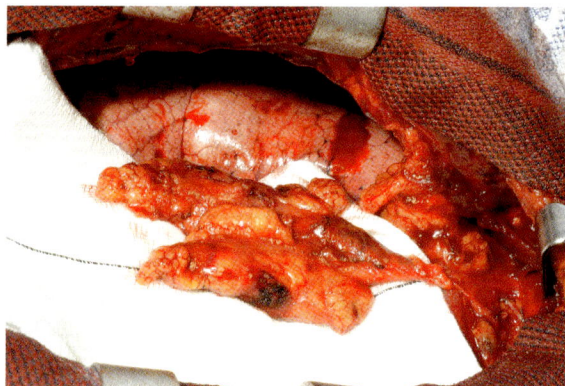

Fig. 9.5 The completely resected thymic specimen from a standard trans-sternal thymectomy on a surgical swab (white material)

gentle traction and division of the thyrothymic ligament (Fig. 9.5).

Variation of the classic trans-sternal thymectomy, such as the partial sternal-splitting technique [33], have been advocated to reduce the degree of surgical invasion and to produce a better cosmetic result. Here, a small skin incision commencing 1.5 cm below the sternal notch is extended to the middle of the sternum at the level of the fourth and fifth rib. The extent of sternal division follows this skin incision or may be limited to splitting the manubrium to the angle of Louis. Retraction of the sternum usually leads to it splitting from the remainder of the body of the sternum at an interspace, and provides good exposure of the anterior mediastinum to perform thymectomy (Fig. 9.6). The sternum can be easily reconstructed at the end of the procedure. Most non-thymomatous MG cases can be resected with this technique, but where there is cervical extension an additional neck incision may be required. This approach, however, is usually inadequate for thymomas.

Extended Trans-sternal Thymectomy

The technique for extended trans-sternal thymectomy begins with the same midline incision and division of the sternum [29]. It differs from the standard thymectomy by actively opening both pleural cavities widely to inspect all the mediastinal structures up to the hilar sites. The phrenic nerves are identified on the lateral aspects of the mediastinal pleura on both sides (Figs 9.7 and 9.8) and preserved bilaterally by careful sharp dissection of the thymic and adipose tissue off the medial aspects of the adjacent pleura (Fig. 9.9). The gland is then removed

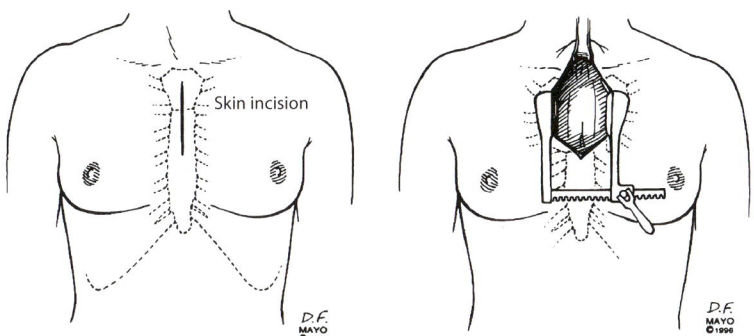

Fig. 9.6 Partial sternal-splitting technique [33] (Used with permission)

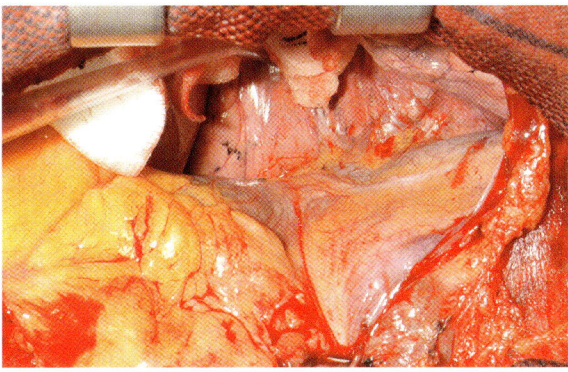

Fig. 9.7 The left phrenic nerve seen on the mediastinal pleura adjacent to the left lung. The white material is a surgical swab.

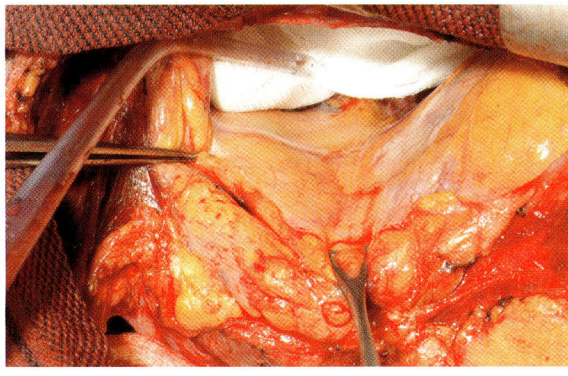

Fig. 9.8 The right phrenic nerve seen on the mediatinal pleura adjacent to the right lung. The white material is a surgical swab.

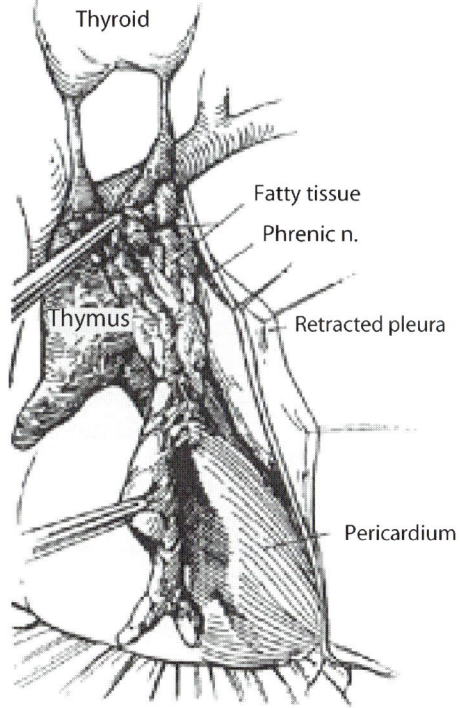

Fig. 9.9 Mobilization of phrenic nerves is of paramount importance to thymectomy [29] (Used with permission)

together with the sheets of mediastinal pleura medial to the phrenic nerves en bloc with the mediastinal fat from the diaphragm caudally to the phrenic nerves laterally and the thyroid gland superiorly (Fig. 9.10). When completed the resection leaves a bare area previously occupied by the anterior and superior mediastinal contents (Fig. 9.11). Extension of the resection to the neck into the retrothyroid area and around the carotid sheath or into the posterior mediastinum around the aortopulmonary window is avoided to reduce the risk of phrenic, vagus and laryngeal nerve damage. It results in a more aggressive mediastinal resection than the standard trans-sternal technique, and it is the authors' current preferred resection strategy.

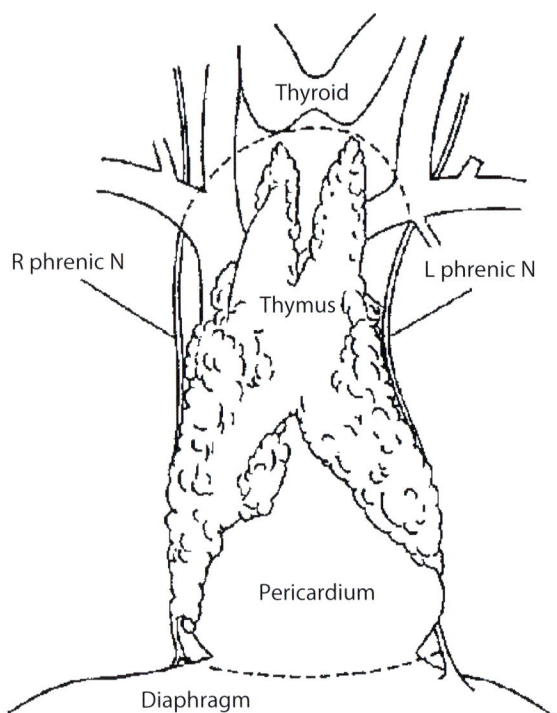

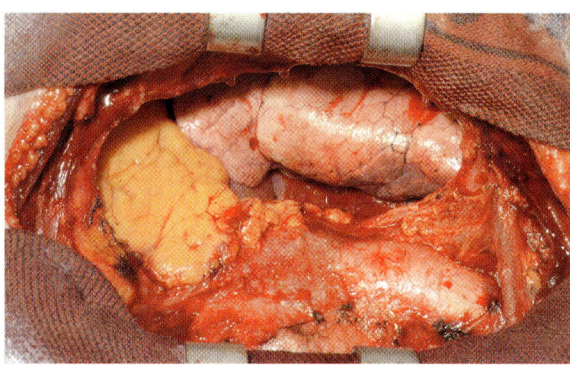

Fig. 9.11 The mediastinal space occupied by the resected thymic specimen

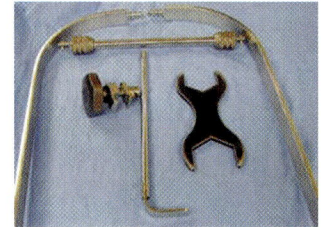

Fig. 9.10 Margins of extended thymectomy. *L* = left, *R* = right, *N* = nerve [68] (Used with permission)

Fig. 9.12 Cooper thymectomy retractor

Transverse Sternal Thymectomy

A short upper transverse sternotomy was described two decades ago as another variation, but failed to find general acceptance [34]. Thymectomy is undertaken through a limited (approximately 15 cm) transverse incision above the sternomanubrial junction, extending into the first intercostal spaces [35]. The transverse sternal approach has also been used with an infra-mammary skin incision (clamshell incision) to obtain good exposure for the radical resection of invasive tumours [36].

Transcervical Thymectomy

This approach offers a less invasive approach to thymectomy in MG patients, as well as the diagnosis and definitive treatment of selected cervical thymic tumours. The trans-cervical approach was first described by Schumacher and Roth in 1912 [37]. Crile in 1966 introduced it for myasthenic patients [12], as did Kirschner [38]. The approach was revived in 1988 by Cooper, along with a specific sternal retractor on the basis that morbidity is minimal [8]. (Cooper Thymectomy Retractor, Pilling Company, Ft. Washington, PA, USA) (Fig. 9.12) [39].

A 4 cm curved incision following the natural lines of the neck is made 2 cm above the sternal notch, centred on the midline. The sternocleidomastoid muscles are divided at their ligamentous insertions to the sternum. The upper lobes of the thymus are identified cephalad to the sternal notch level and freed up from the surrounding tissues. The thymic veins draining deeply to the innominate vein are identified and divided. The sternum is then retracted anteriorly to the point where the patient is almost lifted off the table. This permits the complete removal of the thymus along with all mediastinal fat. Advocates of this technique claim that both sides of the pleural sheets and the aortopulmonary window can be inspected for removal of ectopic thymic or suspicious fatty tissue.

Usually a thymoma is considered to be a contraindication for this technique [18, 40]. Others have, however, reported using it for even patients with thymoma [41], particularly if they are small and non-invasive [40, 42]. In these patients, a complementary sternotomy or mediastinotomy may occasionally be necessary. The limited space between the sternum anteriorly and the innominate vein and mediastinum posteriorly, however, renders difficult the safe dissection and delivery of tumours greater than 4 cm in diameter. Thus, the strategy for the trans-cervical approach for thymic neoplasms should be selective, and also accompanied by a low threshold for extending the incision and converting it to a partial or full sternotomy, so as to avoid compromise on safety or completeness of resection [40].

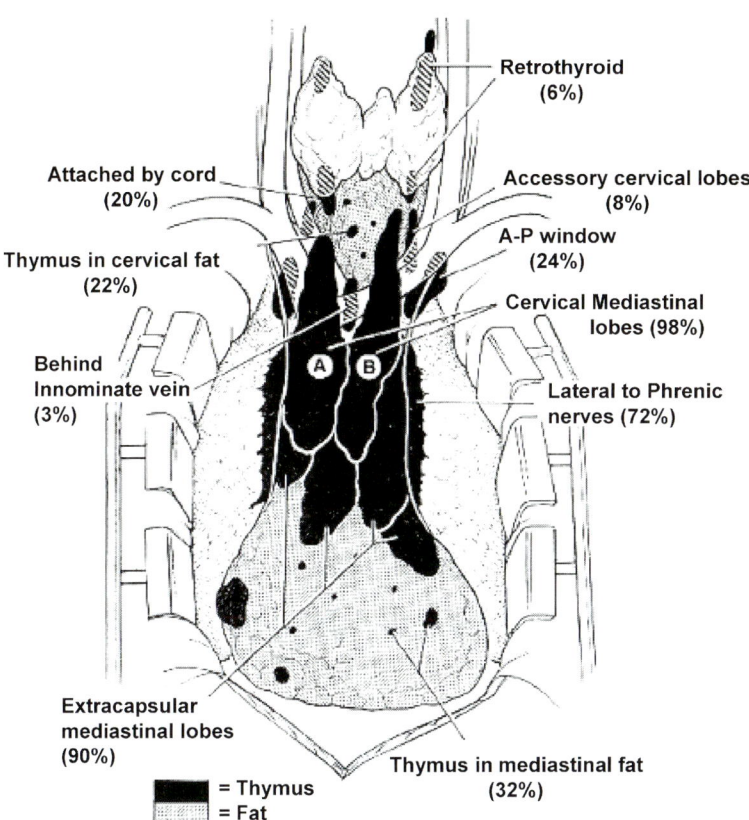

Retrothyroid
(6%)

Attached by cord
(20%)

Thymus in cervical fat
(22%)

Behind
Innominate vein
(3%)

Accessory cervical lobes
(8%)

A-P window
(24%)

Cervical Mediastinal
lobes (98%)

Lateral to Phrenic
nerves (72%)

A   B

Extracapsular
mediastinal lobes
(90%)

Thymus in mediastinal fat
(32%)

= Thymus
= Fat

Fig. 9.13 Composite anatomy of thymus and distribution of thymic tissue to the mediastinum and to the neck. *Black* = thymus, *gray* = fat that may contain islands of thymus and microscopic thymus. *A-P* = aorto-pulmonary window [55] (Used with permission)

This approach has been promoted because it shortens hospital stay, decreases complications and reduces cost [8, 43, 44]. It has been criticised, however, as being technically demanding and difficult to demonstrate.

Maximal Thymectomy

This technique combines trans-sternal thymectomy with cervical exploration for thymic tissue with en bloc removal of thymic tissue. The finding of thymic tissue in pathological specimens and at surgery outside the confines of the classical cervico-mediastinal lobes provides the rationale for this approach, whose goal is the removal of all thymic tissue. Several authors have reported extracapsular thymic tissue [45]. Jaretzki found thymic tissue beyond the thymic lobes in the mediastinum in 98% of patients, and in the neck in 32% of patients, and defined these tissues as a "variation" of normal and not "ectopic" thymic tissue [16] (Fig. 9.13). Residual thymic tissue after thymectomy was identified as being responsible for recurrence of thymic hyperplasia [46]. Removal of as little as 2 g of residual thymic tissue has been shown to result in remission of MG [47]. Jaretzki, in a study of the "estimated" amount of thymic tissue removed by various approaches, suggested differences that favoured maximal thymectomy (as shown previously in Fig. 9.3). These

conclusions are not surprising given the anatomical findings of Jaretzki and Wolff [15], and Fig. 9.13 provides the intellectual foundation for the maximal thymectomy approach. Given the extensive resection there have been concerns regarding the potential for higher morbidity with this approach. In more than 200 maximal thymectomies preformed by Jaretzki, however, there was no report of a nerve injury or of increased incidence of bleeding [48, 49].

A cervical transverse incision 2–3 cm above the sternal notch is combined with a midline incision and a complete median sternotomy [43]. The skin incisions may be combined into a "T" for better exposure in patients with short necks, in reoperations or with large thymomas. All thymic tissue is then removed en bloc with the mediastinal fat. The mediastinal pleural sheets are removed, avoiding damage to the phrenic nerves laterally. Care is also taken to avoid damaging the vagus nerve on the left, as it lies posteriorly and close to the left phrenic nerve, where it gives rise to the recurrent laryngeal nerve at this level. The pericardiophrenic fat and all fatty tissue from the diaphragm to the innominate vein, and from hilum to hilum, are excised (Fig. 9.14). Fat that lies in the sulcus between cava and the ascending aorta on the right, and in the aortopulmonary window on the left, is also removed. The cervical dissection then follows, exploring for thymic tissue posterior and superior to the thyroid

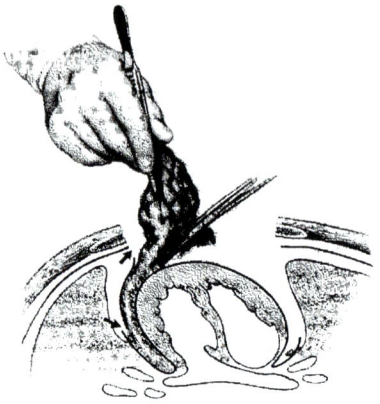

Fig. 9.14 Mobilization and resection of thymus in maximal thymectomy technique: sharp dissection on pericardium; en bloc resection from diaphragm to innominate vein and from hilum to hilum, including fatty thymic tissue in the 'aortopulmonary window' and aortocaval grove, and both sheets of mediastinal pleura. *Arrows* indicate site of both mediatinal pleural incisions on the right. Thymus has been mobilized under the left phrenic nerve [79] (Used with permission)

gland, as well as adjacent to the vagus nerves. Preservation of at least the superior parathyroid glands and avoidance of damage to the recurrent laryngeal nerves at this level is critical [49–51].

VATS (Video-Assisted Thoracic Surgery) Thymectomy

Thoracoscopic thymectomy was first described by Sugarbaker in 1993 [52]. It was promoted on the basis of providing very good exposure and visualization of the anterior mediastinum with enhanced magnification and lighting, and easy access to the lower cervical area for removal of the superior thymic poles, together with minimal invasion and improved cosmesis, less pronounced impairment and faster recovery of pulmonary function, less post-operative pain and shorter in-hospital stay [53, 54]. The main drawback to this approach is its potential for incomplete resection [44, 55, 56]. The possibility of residual thymic remnants in the surrounding fatty tissue with VATS thymectomy [57] has led to concentration on the optimum technique for performing extended thymectomy by thoracoscopy. Approaches from either the left [58] or the right [59] or both sides [60] have been proposed. The right-sided approach allows greater manoeuvrability of instruments in the wider right pleural cavity, and easier identification of the innominate vein [61] and definition of the venous anatomy [62]. The left-sided approach is reported to permit safer dissection (as the superior vena cava lies outside of the surgical field) and extensive removal of the perithymic fatty tissue from the left pericardiophrenic angle and the aortopulmonary window. Cardiomegaly, however, may limit exposure of the gland [57, 63]. With a unilateral approach, moreover, dissection of the pericardial adipose tissue on the opposite side is always a problem [61, 64] and has led to the use of the bilateral thoracoscopic technique [59].

The patient is anaesthetised with a double-lumen endotracheal tube for one-lung ventilation and placed in a 45-degree off-centre position. Four flexible trocars are inserted into the hemithorax (Fig. 9.15). Introduction of a pneumomediastinum facilitates resection [65]. One-

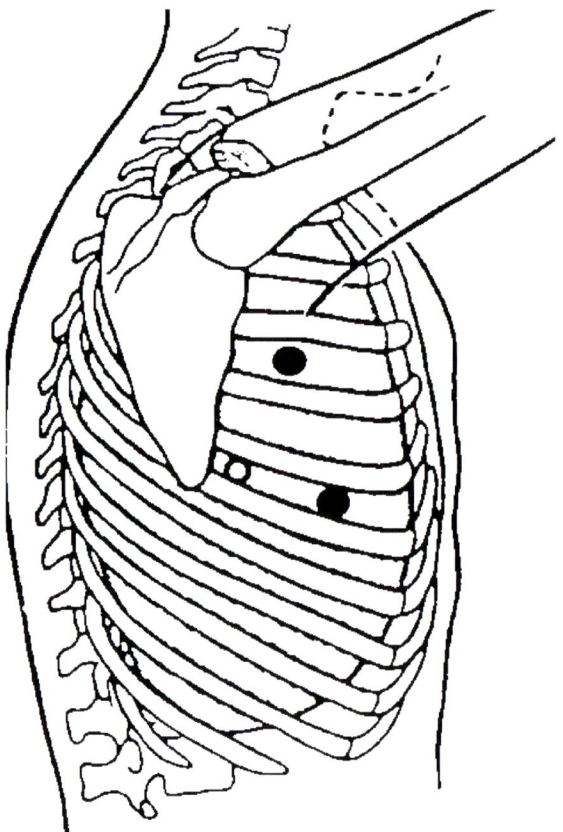

Fig. 9.15 VATS resection: Positions of camera and instrument ports for right sided VATS thymectomy [67] (Used with permission)

lung ventilation is used intermittently to aid access, and bronchial secretions are frequently aspirated to reduce the risk of post-operative atelectasis. The entire gland and all mediastinal perithymic fatty tissues are removed, and the surgical specimen is extracted through an endoscopic specimen bag with a drainage tube left in situ in the anterior mediastinum. There are also descriptions of modifications of the standard VATS technique, such as the use of a video-assisted infra-mammary cosmetic incision [66].

Thymectomy Results

Analysing results from thymectomy studies is not without problems. Data derived from some of these studies are evidence-based medicine class II. Others are class III or less. Data from standard trans-sternal thymectomy results in MG are limited; complete remission rates of up to 32% in a 10-year period have been reported [8]. The results for extended thymectomy are more readily available, and with follow-up from 3 to 13 or 15 years, complete remission rates from 26% to 67%, and clinical improvement rates from 58% to 94% have been reported [10, 27, 29, 68–76]. Masaoka et al. reported a remission rate of 45.8% at 5 years, 55.7% at 10 years and 67.2% at 15 years, while their improvement rate was about 90% at 3 years and plateaued thereafter. In the same series, remission of MG in patients with thymoma reached 32.4% in 3 years and improvement was 82.5% in 1 year, which then also plateaued (Fig. 9.16) [68]. With trans-cervical thymectomy, complete remission and clinical improvement at a follow-up period of up to 8.4 years was 35–44% and 81–85% respectively [43, 44, 77]. There is, nevertheless,

concern about the ability for radical thymectomy with this approach, as residual thymus was found in all reoperated patients (4.3%) of a series after trans-cervical thymectomy [78].

Bulkley et al. [19] reported that extended cervico-mediastinal thymectomy was associated with a greater than two-fold chance of improvement, compared to conventional trans-sternal thymectomy, and suggests that prediction or identification pre-operatively of ectopic thymic tissue could usefully determine the appropriate surgical approach. This, however, is not currently achievable. For persistent or recurrent severe symptoms after previous trans-cervical or sub-maximal trans-sternal resection, re-operation by maximal thymectomy is recommended [79]. Maximal thymectomy results in 20–46% remission and 86–97% improvement at 10-year follow-up [16, 18, 19, 55, 80]. This approach reflects the chance of avoiding thymic remnants after surgery, which Jaretzki described as 98–100% in maximal thymectomy, 85–95% in extended thymectomy, 75–80% in modified trans-cervical thymectomy, 70–75% in trans-sternal thymectomy, and 40–50% in simple trans-cervical thymectomy [55]. The clinical sig-

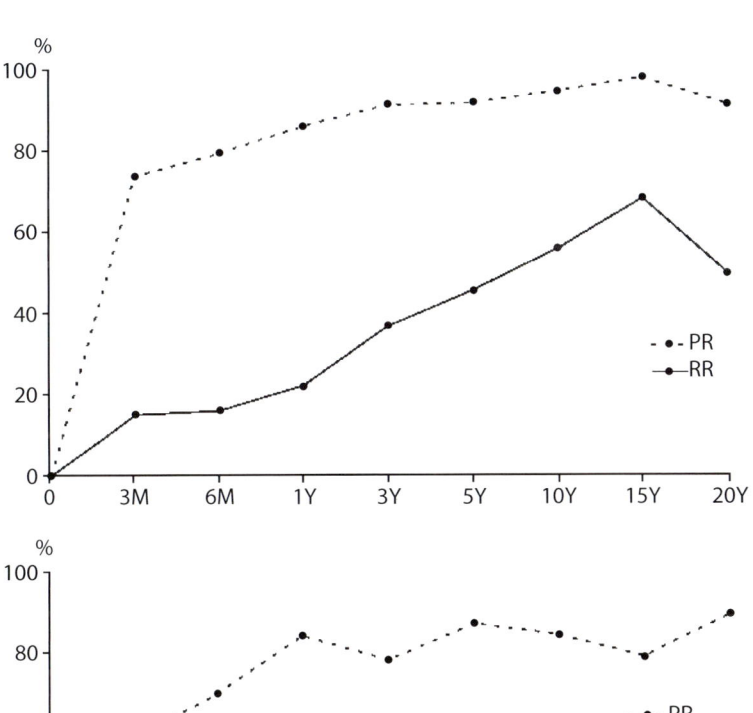

Fig. 9.16 Outcome in patients with non-thymomatous MG (upper graph) and with thymomatous MG (lower graph) following extended trans-sternal thymectomy. *PR* = palliation rate, *RR* = remission rate [68] (Used with permission)

nificance of ectopic thyroid tissue is reflected by Ashour [47], who reported in a follow-up of 14.5 months following maximal thymectomy that the remission rate was 13.3% in patients with ectopic thymic tissue and 47.8% in patients with no ectopic thymic tissue; the improvement rate was 66.6% in the former group and 100% in the latter.

Figures 9.17 and 9.18 show the comparative remission rates after cervical thymectomy, and the different sternal thymectomy approaches for non-thymomatous MG. Jaretzki [55] emphasized that crude data is not statistically acceptable, hence life-table analyses using Kaplan–Meier curves must be used for comparison of the results (see Chap. 13).

VATS thymectomy has shown a 14–50% remission rate and a 83–96% improvement rate at up to 2–6 years follow-up [56, 58, 61, 81, 82]. Thus, it is suggested that VATS thymectomy is as effective in the management of MG in non-thymomatous patients or stage I non-invasive thymomas as traditional open surgical approaches, and has led to the development of a substantial lobby for early thymectomy in MG patients because of its improved cosmetic result [61].

Table 9.1 describes the outcomes from 21 cohorts of patients from 1953 until 1998 [83]. In summary, complete remission has been reported in 20–50%, clinical improvement in 54–97%, an unchanged condition in 4–18% and deterioration of the disease in 2–11% of the MG patients that underwent thymectomy [18, 19, 28, 36, 55, 68, 70, 79, 84–86]. Comparison of the different approaches to thymectomy and extraction of unbiased results is difficult because of the heterogeneous manner of presentation of data (patient exclusion criteria, classification systems, definition of improvement or remission, statistical analysis methods, etc.). The greatest variation is in the description of the post-operative clinical status of the patients. DeFilippi et al. have suggested that surgical outcome is graded according to the following criteria: complete remission of all medication, asymptomatic on decreased medication, improved with decreased medication, no change, and worsening symptoms [77]. This was one of up to 15 clinical classifications that were offered at that time. As a result of this absence of agreement the Medical Scientific Advisory Board (MSAB) of the Myasthenia Gravis Foundation of America (MGFA) formed a task Force to

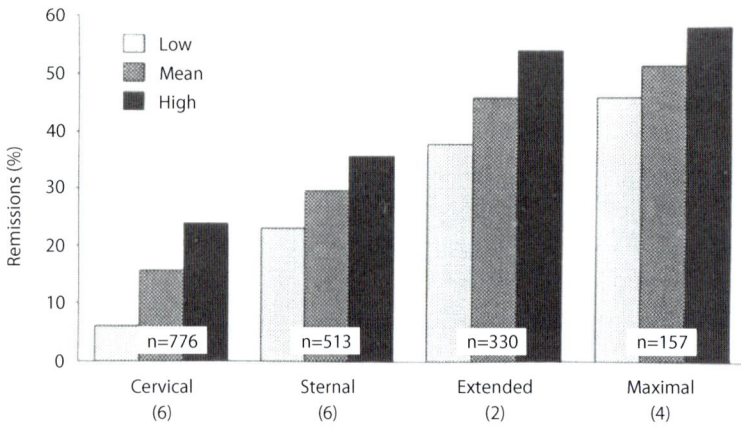

Fig. 9.17 Comparative remission rates for MG with no thymoma (uncorrected). Collated from 18 reports (6 transcervical, 6 transsternal, 2 extended and 4 maximal thymectomies). The difference between the maximal and the cervical procedures is highly significant (p = 0.00001) [79] (Used with permission)

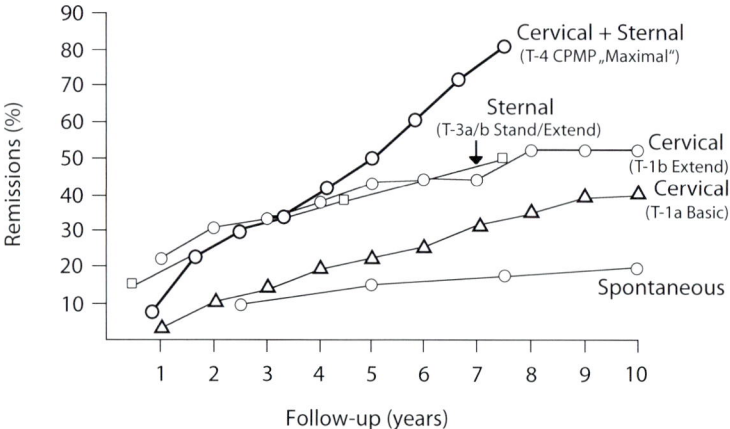

Fig. 9.18 Remission rates (life-table analysis) after four thymectomy techniques for non-thymomatous myasthenia gravis. Cervical + Sternal = T-4 CPMC ("Maximal" thymectomy); Sternal = T-3a/b (Stand/Extend: more extensive than the standard transsternal thymectomy / T-3a, but less extensive than the aggressive extended transsternal thymectomy / T-3b); Cervical = T-1b Extend ("extended" transcervical thymectomy); Cervical = T-1a (Basic transcervical thymectomy); Spontaneous = spontaneous remissions in children [92] (Used with permission)

Table 9.1 Thymectomy for MG outcome by cohort survey – a review of the literature. [From Gronseth GS, Barohn RJ (2000) Practice parameter: thymectomy for autoimmune myasthenia gravis (an evidence-based review). Report of the Quality Standards Subcommittee of the American Academy of Neurology. Neurology 55:7–15]

Author (year)	MF remission				Asymptomatic				Improved				Survived			
	NH %	TH %	RR	CI	NH %	TH %	RR	CI	NH %	TH %	RR	CI	NH %	TH %	RR	CI
Christensen et al. (1998)	–	–	–	–	–	–	–	–	–	–	–	–	56	84	1.5	1.3–1.8
Evoli et al. (1998)	10	33	3.3	–	–	–	–	–	–	–	–	–	–	–	–	–
Beekman et al. (1997)	25	35	1.4	0.7–2.7	43	49	0.9	0.5–1.5	80	96	1.2	1.0–1.4	–	–	–	–
Werneck et al. (1996)	50	25	0.5	0.2–1.0	60	54	0.9	0.6–1.4	100	87	0.87	0.75–1.0	100	90	0.9	0.8–1.0
Evoli et al. (1996)	7.7	7.7	1.0	0.2–4.4	–	–	–	–	–	–	–	–	–	–	–	–
Beghi et al. (1991)	8.0	17	2.1	1.2–3.8	–	–	–	–	–	–	–	–	–	–	–	–
Mantegazza et al. (1990)	6.1	13	2.2	1.3–3.4	24	38	1.6	1.3–2.0	–	–	–	–	–	–	–	–
Donaldson et al. (1990)	8.8	26	3.0	1.2–7.2	28	62	2.2	1.4–3.4	–	–	–	–	–	–	–	–
Papatestas et al. (1987)	–	–	–	–	14	22	1.6	1.4–2.0	–	–	–	–	76	91	1.2	1.1–1.2
Grob et al. (1987)	–	–	–	–	11	7.7	0.7	0.–1.1	49	44	0.9	0.8–1.1	85	51	0.6	0.5–0.6
Scadding et al. (1985)	11	25	2.3	1.0–5.4	–	–	–	–	27	70	2.6	1.6–4.2	–	–	–	–
Rodriguez et al. (1983)	34	48	1.4	1.0–2.2	–	–	–	–	63	82	1.3	1.0–1.6	84	92	1.1	1.0–1.2
Oosterhuis et al. (1981)	–	–	–	–	20	26	1.3	0.9–1.9	–	–	–	–	95	95	1.0	1.0–1.1
Buckingham et al. (1976)	7.5	34	4.5	2.0–10	–	–	–	–	24	67	2.8	1.8–4.3	58	87	1.5	1.2–1.8
Emeryk, Strugalsa (1976)	9.3	23	2.5	1.1–5.4	–	–	–	–	56	62	1.1	0.8–1.4	83	91	1.1	1.0–1.2
Perlo et al. (1971)	–	–	–	–	17	41	2.4	1.8–3.1	28	90	3.2	2.7–3.7	–	–	–	–
Zeldowicz, Saxton (1969)	–	–	–	–	27	84	3.1	1.7–5.8	50	95	1.9	1.3–2.8	90	99	1.1	1.0–1.3
Henson et al. (1965)	26	52	2.0	1.1–3.6	36	65	1.8	1.1–2.8	36	65	1.8	1.2–3.9	96	86	0.9	0.8–1.1
Simpson (1958)	16	21	1.3	0.8–2.2	21	34	1.6	1.1–2.4	33	56	1.7	1.3–2.3	75	83	1.1	1.0–1.3
Eaton, Clagett (1955)	6.2	17	2.7	1.2–6.1	–	–	–	–	33	66	2.0	1.5–2.6	73	88	1.2	1.0–1.4
Eaton et al. (1953)	10	18	1.8	0.6–4.9	–	–	–	–	44	70	1.6	1.1–2.3	85	94	1.1	1.0–1.3

develop a series of classifications for the post-intervention status of a patient, which is now in common usage [87]: complete remission, pharmacologic remission, minimal manifestations, improved, unchanged, worse, exacerbation and death. In general, complete remission and clinical improvement are the most used follow-up parameters in the literature, and were used in the authors' own series.

The mortality from thymectomy is 0–2% [19, 28, 36, 68, 70, 74, 76, 85, 86, 88–92]. Morbidity ranges from 4% to 33% [19, 28, 40, 44, 70, 72, 92, 93]. This variation is probably again the result of the differences in the definition of morbidity in each of the series, which may report minor or major morbidity, as reflected by the widely varying incidence of post-operative pneumonia described below. The specific complications described after thymectomy are: retention of respiratory secretions (10%) [94,95], lung atelectasis (7%) [94, 95], pneumonia (1–4%) [19, 28, 70, 72, 76, 90] or as high as 14.4% [88], wound infection 1–7% [19, 70, 76, 88–92], hydrothorax (4–4.5%) [19, 76], injury to the phrenic nerve (0–4.5%) [19, 70, 89, 90, 92, 96], damage to the recurrent laryngeal nerve (0–4.5%) [19, 56, 85, 92], sternal dehiscence (1–4%) [90, 92, 93], tracheal injury (3.5%) [97], pneumothorax (2%) [76], cardiac arrhythmias (1–2%) [76, 88, 94], mediastinitis (1.6%) [88], anaemia requiring transfusion (1%) [19], thoracic empyema (1%) [92], pulmonary embolism (1%) [19, 28, 92], deep venous thrombosis (1%) [76], subclavian vein thrombosis (1%) [76], chylothorax (0.5–1%) [19, 92], and bleeding (0.5%) [19]. The major general complication, therefore, is respiratory insufficiency, which may occur in as many as 24% of elderly patients [27]. If the patient's condition does not improve, re-intubation for pronounced myasthenic muscle weakness or abundant respiratory secretions and subsequent tracheostomy may occur in as many as 6% of this group [85]. A similar scenario may also arise from laryngeal nerve damage intra-operatively. The response to these complications is also heterogeneous, with the rate of tracheostomy varying among the series from 0% up to 100% [42, 76, 90, 95, 97, 98].

Prognostic Factors of Thymectomy Outcome

A number of factors have been identified as having an influence on prognosis after thymectomy.

Clinical Outcome over Time

The delayed effect after thymectomy for MG is well described. Most patients respond within six months to one year after surgery rather than in the immediate post-operative period, but this response is sustained for at least a 10-year period thereafter [19, 92]. Remission increases slowly over time [77, 99], ranging from 1–13% at 1 year, 8–36% at 3 and 5 years [58, 106] and up to 62% at >7 years [16]. Masaoka et al. [68], in a 20-year follow-

up of their patients, found that the remission rate of the non-thymomatous patients was 45.8% at 5 years, 55.7% at 10 years, 67.2% at 15 years and 50.0% at 20 years, while in thymomatous patients the remission rate was 23.0% at 5 years, 30.0% at 10 years, 31.8% at 15 years and 37.5% at 20 years. The improvement rate similarly increased from 59% at 1 year to 83–96% at 5–10 years [19, 58]. Others, however, did not find the duration of follow-up to be a significant factor in assessing improvement [101]. This delayed response is difficult to explain. It is possible that the disease process continues early after surgery because of deposits of previously exported immune components at extra-thymic sites, which gradually decay with time.

Thymectomy and Pathology of the Thymus

Many have reported that thymic histology does not influence outcome after thymectomy [19, 60, 86, 100–102, 106]; others have reported that histology did appreciably influence the effect of surgery [67, 90, 103]. The presence of thymic hyperplasia more significantly increased the chance of complete remission [28, 82, 96, 99–102], although a few have not substantiated this [16,28]. Others found that absence of thymoma favoured outcome [16, 28, 36, 67, 68, 102, 103, 107, 108, 119], but again a few studies failed to confirm these findings [104, 105]. The presence of germinal centres in the gland, a reflection of thymic activity, positively influenced outcome [98, 114]. The delay in the onset of remission post-thymectomy was proportional to the number and activity of the germinal centres [106] (Fig. 9.19) and may support the previously stated hypothesis that the delay could be influenced by the presence of extra-thymic deposits of immunological agents.

Duration of the Disease

There is evidence that a shorter duration of symptoms pre-operatively favours outcome [10, 36, 42, 58, 68, 69, 72, 103, 107, 108]. Thus, there are reports that results were better when the duration of disease was 12 months or less [58, 77, 103, 106, 108, 109], and it is possible that this effect is independent of the severity of disease. Surgery early after the onset of MG may be essential to prevent the substantial export of autoreactive T cells from the thymus to extra-thymic organs. This appears to be the case with MG due to thymitis [110]. Others, however, have failed to confirm that duration of the disease before thymectomy is not a significant factor in outcome after MG [75, 90, 99–102].

Thymectomy and Age

Perlo et al. [111] found no or only involuted thymic tissue microscopically in autopsies of thymuses from patients

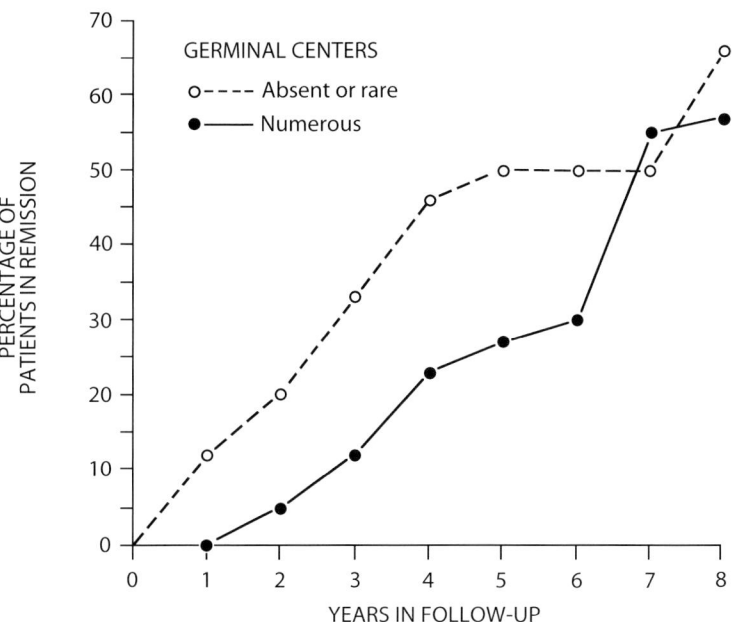

Fig. 9.19 MG remission after thymectomy in relation to germinal centres [106] (Used with permission)

older than 60 years. This has led many to recommend that thymectomy be avoided in the elderly. The literature regarding age as a prognostic factor for the outcome after thymectomy in MG is, however, conflicting. Some studies show age as not being a significant factor in outcome [16, 19, 58, 71, 75, 90, 99, 100, 101–102], while others show that younger age favoured a better outcome [36, 68, 69, 72, 112, 113]. The age limit for better outcome with thymectomy has not been established; thymectomy is suggested by some for patients younger than 40 years [86, 103], by others for patients younger than 50 years [28, 114] and by yet others in patients younger than 60 years [27, 115]. Those who advocate thymectomy in all age groups do so on the basis that thymectomy is a safe and effective treatment in the elderly. They also challenge the notion of complete involution of the thymus in this age group. Tscuchida et al. [27], for example, found that thymic hyperplasia was not only present in 45% of the young group, but also in 16% of the older group. Remission and improvement were 40% and 57% in the younger group, and 8%, but also 75%, in the elderly group, respectively. Juvenile patients experience remission of the disease more frequently than adults [116]. Thymectomy at these ages should, therefore, be considered only after prolonged medical therapy [9]. In line with adult patients, some have recommended that thymectomy should be considered at the onset of juvenile generalised MG [109, 117, 118], using video-assisted thoracoscopic techniques [119, 120].

Thymectomy and Stage of Myasthenia

Patients with mild generalised MG symptoms treated with thymectomy achieved remission more frequently in many series [42, 50, 68, 69, 72, 101, 103, 106]. Stage of the disease had no effect on outcome in others [28, 58, 77, 90].

Medication

High pyridostigmine dose is reported to predict worse outcome after thymectomy [108], although this effect of the pre-operative patients' medication on surgical outcome was not confirmed by others [100, 102].

Thymectomy and Gender

There are conflicting results in the literature on the influence of gender on outcome. Some show no influence on outcome [10, 16, 58, 86, 90, 121–124], while others report that female MG patients are more likely to benefit from thymectomy [10, 68, 69, 72, 75, 125].

Thymectomy and Antibody Status

Despite the fact that 87% of patients with generalised MG are seropositive for anti-acetylcholine receptor antibodies

[126], pre-operative antibody titre to acetylcholine receptors and post-operative change in titre antibody status have not been shown to effect outcome after thymectomy [16, 90, 101].

Refractory Myasthenia

In general, the failure of a surgical procedure to achieve its goal, such as symptomatic relief, is associated with inadequate surgery, be it resection, reconstruction, replacement or revascularisation. This may also be the case with thymectomy for MG, where incomplete resection may affect outcome. Residual thymic tissue was found at the completion of VATS thymectomy in all patients who showed no benefit from initial transcervical thymectomy [127, 128]. Ectopic thymic tissue was considered an unfavourable prognostic factor by Ashour, who hypothesised that it might indicate the presence of additional covert ectopic sites [47]. Thus, in refractory myasthenia a thorough search by imaging, which is usually only profitable with thymomas and operative exploration of mediastinal and cervical structures, must be performed. There is a special relevance for this in non-thymomatous MG, where there are reports of primary thymomas arising from residual ectopic thymic tissues following thymectomy [129, 130] (see also Maximal Thymectomy section, above).

This may not, however, be the only explanation for surgical refractoriness. The disease process at least in the early post-operative period may not be governed by the thymus alone. Extra-thymic deposits of T cells exported prior to resection may continue to exercise an effect after thymic resection. If confirmed, this has significant implications for the surgical strategy of managing MG.

Re-operations

The aim of re-operation in MG patients is to complete an otherwise incomplete thymectomy [131]. As described above, refractory myasthenia or recurrence of symptoms may be due to residual thymic tissue, which is reported in 64–100% of patients who undergo a completion procedure [46, 132]. In the case of the second operation, technical difficulties due to adhesions, and increased risk of wound healing due to high doses of steroids, are relevant [128, 131]. These patients, furthermore, are difficult to manage and complete remission is usually not successful. Despite these limitations and risks, results from surgery are good, and a 75–100% symptomatic improvement has been reported [92, 128, 133]. Thus, in the 10–15% of patients who fail to respond to thymectomy, re-exploration is indicated when a patient shows signs of progressive deterioration of symptoms, particularly after a prolonged and sustained improvement [39]. This recommendation holds even with inconclusive or normal post-operative

CT or MRI imaging, which is usual, with decision-making being based on clinical assessment and evaluation of the extent of the original operation [16, 133].

Thymectomy for Thymoma

Thymomas have been discussed in Chaps. 4 and 7. The therapeutic strategy of thymoma depends on the characteristics of the tumour (invasiveness, resectability and pathologic type). Current treatment guidelines are comprised of complete surgical resection and of multimodality therapy with adjuvant radiotherapy or chemotherapy, or both for patients with advanced disease [134, 135]. Surgery remains the principal treatment.

In line with the general principles of all oncology surgery, thymectomy aims for resection with margins clear of tumour. Thus, where there is direct thymoma involvement or invasion of adjacent structures, successful surgery mandates a wide resection. The pericardium is opened when necessary, and the involved pericardium is resected. Rarely does the tumour invade heart or great vessels. Here the tumour is usually inoperable, but resection may be possible on cardiopulmonary bypass. The pleurae, if involved, are opened and resected. Invasion of the lung could lead to appropriate lung resection, usually as a wedge. Invasion of a phrenic nerve requires its sacrifice so long as the contralateral nerve is preserved. In a cephalic direction a partial thyroidectomy may be necessary. It is essential that all surgery be accompanied by a careful description and the marking of the surgical margins with radiologically visible surgical clips. Finally, a careful microscopic pathological examination is essential to determine the need for adjuvant therapeutic modalities.

Surgery is usually curative in early stage disease [135, 136]. Thus, patients with stage I disease require no further therapy after complete surgical resection, and have a 90–100% 5-year survival rate, and up to an 86% 10-year survival rate [137–140]. Survival for stage II is also good (85% in 5 years and 78% in 10 years) [140, 141]. Overall survival rates after thymectomy for thymoma in the literature are 67–88% in 5 years, 53–81% in 10 years, and up to as high as 86–99% 10-year survival in patients with early stages treated disease and complete resection [22, 137, 142, 143–145]. Moreover, other studies have shown lower rates of overall survival, probably due to advanced stages of treating tumours: 59% 5-year and 34% 10-year survival [146] rates, although up to 33% survival rates at 25 years has been reported [143].

The major prognostic factors for long-term survival in thymoma patients are the pathological stage of the tumour [21, 86, 137, 146–148], the completeness of resection [21, 137, 141, 143, 146, 148, 149] and the histology [137, 149, 150] (Fig. 9.20). Significant correlation has been demonstrated between the absence and presence of great vessel invasion, and between the presence of in-

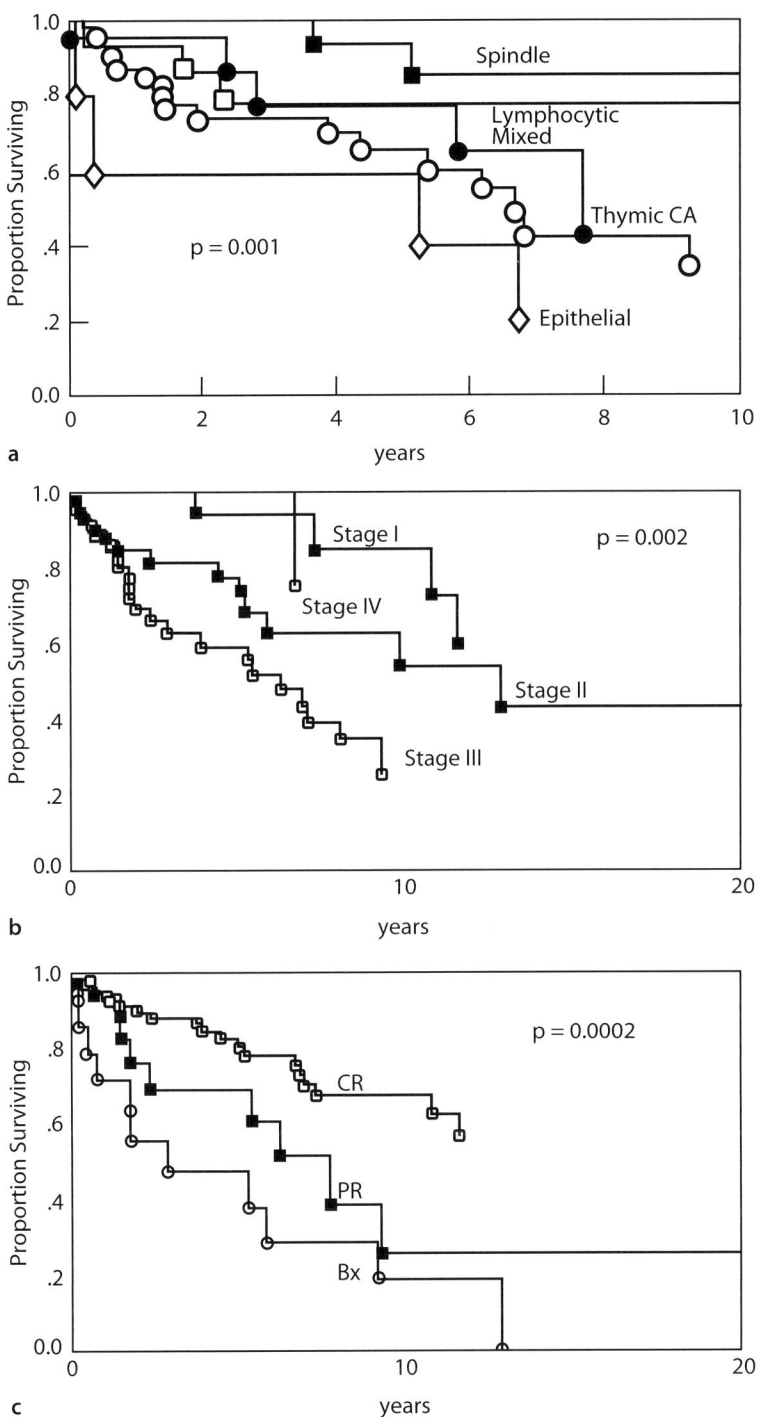

Fig. 9.20 Thymectomy outcome in patients with thymoma: **a** survival by histology, **b** survival by Masaoka staging system, **c** survival by extent of surgical resection (*CR* = complete resection, *PR* = partial resection, *Bx* = biopsy) [137] (Used with permission)

vasion of structures other than the great vessels and the presence of great vessel invasion. Histologically, epithelial cell type predominance increases with clinical stage [149]. Medullary and mixed thymomas are, therefore, considered to be benign tumours with no risk of recurrence, even when capsular invasion is present. Organoid and cortical thymomas show intermediate invasiveness, while well-differentiated thymic carcinomas are generally invasive and have a significantly increased risk of relapse and death, even in stage II patients [151].

The relationship of thymoma with MG further confounds the issue of surgical results. The presence of MG was proposed as a prognostic factor for poor outcome [152], but more recent studies failed to demonstrate this [144, 148, 153–156]. Well-differentiated thymic carcinoma histology, age of more than 55 years, and interval from the onset of symptoms to thymectomy of less than one year were found to be independent predictors of non-remission of MG after thymectomy for thymoma [157]. Thymoma is associated with the occurrence of other extra-thymic malignancy (lung, GI tract, liver and breast cancer) and some evidence exists that thymectomy may inhibit the expression of this relationship [158].

The operative mortality for thymectomy in thymoma patients with MG is 1.4–5% [86, 141]. Remission of myasthenic symptoms occurs in about 15% (higher in stage I tumours) and improvement in about 60% of patients [86] (Fig. 9.10). Success in terms of remission and improvement with early thymectomy for non-thymoma MG was described above on the basis that early surgery prevents the substantial export of autoreactive T cells to extra-thymic organs. This temporal relationship does not exist with thymectomy for MG associated with thymoma. This may be because the dissemination of autoreactive T cells to extra-thymic sites has occurred for some time before the emergence of myasthenic symptoms. Thymectomy for thymoma is, therefore, mainly for oncological purposes and control of local complications. It is less successful at alleviating MG [117].

Thymoma grows slowly. Recurrences occur in 10–30% of patients after complete resection, and may progress slowly even in the absence of treatment [137, 141, 147, 159–161]. The recurrence rate at 10 years has been reported as 40% elsewhere [137]. The stage of disease is the only identified independent prognostic factor for recurrence [137]. Recurrence is usually local in the pleural space. Systemic (haematogenous, lymphatic) metastasis, unlike with other carcinomas, is uncommon [162]. Recurrence after resection of stage I or II thymomas is usually local. In stage III or IV thymomas, while pleural, pericardial or pulmonary metastases are found, metastatic recurrence may also occur farther afield [163]. These loco-regional metastases are thought to result from malignant implants related to thymoma capsular disruption, secondary either to tumour growth or to surgical resection. Re-resection in recurrent thymomas is recommended [86, 141, 159, 164] for patients with limited spread, where complete resection is feasible [162]. Survival after re-resection for recurrent thymoma is 37–70% at 5 years and 16–43% at 10 years [86, 162, 163] (Fig. 9.21). Long-term survival, therefore, is possible even with resection for recurrent thymoma [164].

Thymectomy for Thymoma and Adjuvant Therapy

As discussed above, recurrence of thymoma is related to residual tumour, which is often microscopic [153]. Thus, although surgery is the gold standard for thymoma [163], adjuvant therapy in the form chemotherapy and radiotherapy plays a potentially important role and is discussed in later chapters.

Thymectomy for Myasthenia Gravis – the Oxford Experience

The authors' view is that patients with well-controlled symptoms by medical managements are not suitable can-

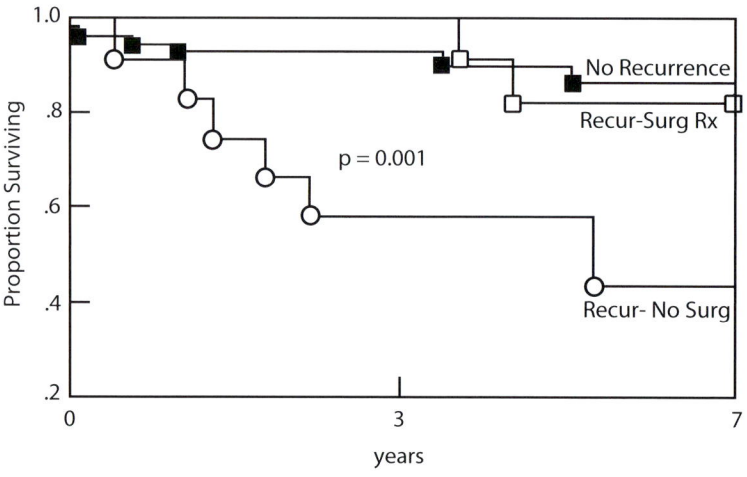

Fig. 9.21 Thymectomy outcome in patients with thymoma – survival of patients with no recurrence, those with recurrence treated by surgical resection and those with recurrence not treated surgically [137] (Used with permission)

didates for thymectomy, as their prognosis is in general good. Candidates for thymectomy, therefore, are patients with symptoms refractory to medical therapy, patients with advanced stages of the disease and patients with thymoma.

In a retrospective review of the Oxford patients over the last decade [165], 85 consecutive patients (65 females; mean age 30.5 years) were enrolled. In terms of pathology, thymoma was present in 11%, hyperplasia in 60% and a normal thymus was found in 29% of the patients. The mean follow-up of the patients was 4.5 ± 3.4 years (range 1–14 years), which represented a total of 376 follow-up years. Extended trans-sternal thymectomy was employed as a standard technique.

There was no mortality in the post-operative period or during the follow-up period. The mean ventilation time was 2.4 ± 7.6 days (range 0–61 days). The mean intensive care stay was 3.2 ± 7.4 days (range 0–58 days) and mean in-hospital stay was 10.2 ± 9.6 days (range 3–75 days). Cumulative early or late morbidity was 16.5%. At the end of the follow-up, 17% of the patients were in complete remission (defined as absence of symptoms and on no anti-myasthenic treatment), 79% reported clinical improvement, and 63% were asymptomatic or in stage I undergoing no or only minimal treatment. Older age was a risk factor for thymic pathology, especially thymoma. The presence of hyperplasia or thymoma did not predict clinical improvement or remission after surgery. A raised anti-acetylcholine receptor antibody titre was found in 93% of patients, but neither the rise nor the value of the titre (the severity of the rise) predicted post-operative remission or symptomatic improvement after surgery. Neither gender nor age were significant prognostic factors of post-operative clinical improvement or remission. Duration of symptoms did not predict outcome, but severity of pre-operative symptoms strongly influenced operative results. Patients with greater severity of symptoms prior to surgery were associated with a greater subsequent improvement. Remission at one year predicted remission at the end of follow-up (Fig. 9.22).

References

1. Sauerbruch F. Mitteilungen aus den Grenzgebieten der Medizin und Chirurgie 1913;25:746.
2. Blalock A, Mason MF, Morgan HG, et al. Myasthenia gravis and tumors of the thymic region. Ann Surg 1939;110:544–561.
3. Blalock A, Harvey A, Ford F, Lilienthal, J Jr. The treatment of myasthenia gravis by removal of the thymus gland. JAMA 1941;117:1529–1531.
4. Blalock A. Thymectomy in the treatment of myasthenia gravis. J Thorac Surg 1944;13:316.
5. Keynes G. The results of thymectomy in myasthenia gravis. Br Med J 1949;2:611–616.
6. Eaton LM, Clagett OT. Thymectomy in the treatment of myasthenia gravis. JAMA 1950;19:963–967.
7. Castleman B. The pathology of the thymus gland in myasthenia gravis. Ann NY Acad Sci 1966;135:496–503.
8. Papatestas AE, Genkins G, Kornfeld P, et al. Effects of thymectomy in myasthenia gravis. Ann Surg 1987;206:79–88.
9. Urschel JD, Grewal RP. Thymectomy for myasthenia gravis. Postgrad Med J 1998;74:139–144.
10. Nieto IP, Robledo JP, Pajuelo MC, et al. Prognostic factors for myasthenia gravis treated by thymectomy: review of 61 cases. Ann Thorac Surg 1999;67:1568–1571.
11. Sanders DB, Kaminski HJ, Jaretzki A III, Phillips LH II, the Evaluation Standards Review Committee, Medical Advisory Board, Myasthenia Gravis Foundation of America. Thymectomy for myasthenia gravis in older patients. J Am Coll Surg 2001;193:340–341.
12. Crile G Jr. Thymectomy through the neck. Surgery 1966;59:213–215.
13. Kirschner PA, Osserman KE, Kark AE. Studies in myasthenia gravis. Transcervical total thymectomy. JAMA 1969;209:906–910.
14. Masaoka A, Nagaoka Y, Kotake Y. Distribution of thymic tissue at the anterior mediastinum. Current procedures in thymectomy. J Thorac Cardiovasc Surg 1975;70:747–754.
15. Jaretzki A 3rd, Bethea M, Wolff M, et al. A rational approach to total thymectomy in the treatment of myasthenia gravis. Ann Thorac Surg 1977;24:120–130.
16. Jaretzki A III, Wolff M. "Maximal" thymectomy for myasthenia gravis. Surgical anatomy and operative technique. J Thorac Cardiovasc Surg 1988;96:711–716.
17. Buckingham JM, Howard FM Jr, Bernatz PE, et al. The value of thymectomy in myasthenia gravis: a computer-assisted matched study. Ann Surg 1976;184:453–458.
18. Ferguson MK. Transcervical thymectomy. Semin Thorac Cardiovasc Surg 1999;11:59–64.
19. Bulkley GB, Bass KN, Stephenson GR et al. Extended cervicomediastinal thymectomy in the integrated management of myasthenia gravis. Ann Surg 1997;226:324–334.

Remission (%)

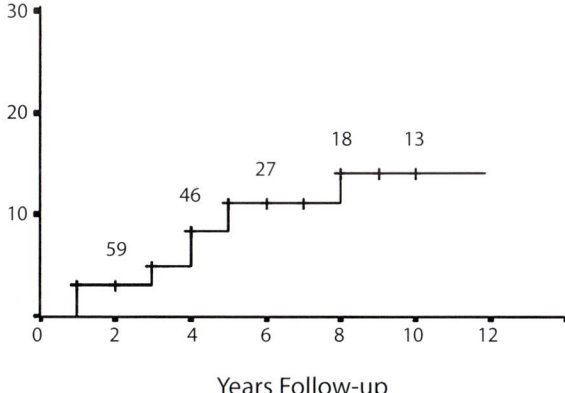

Years Follow-up

Fig. 9.22 Complete stable remission rate after trans-sternal thymectomy [165] (Used with permission)

20. Wilkins KB, Bulkley GB. Thymectomy in the integrated management of myasthenia gravis. Adv Surg 1999;32:105–133.

21. Moore KH, McKenzie PR, Kennedy CW, McCaughan BC. Thymoma: trends over time. Ann Thorac Surg 2001;72:203–207.

22. Jaretzki A, Steinglass KM, Sonett JR. Thymectomy in the management of myasthenia gravis. Semin Neurol 2004;24:49–62.

23. Lanska DJ. Indication for thymectomy in myasthenia gravis. Neurology 1990;40:1828–1829.

24. Roberts PF, Venuta F, Rendina E, et al. Thymectomy in the treatment of ocular myasthenia gravis. J Thorac Cardiovasc Surg 2001;122:562–568.

25. Evoli A, Batocchi AP, Minisci C, Di Schino C, Tonali P. Therapeutic options in ocular myasthenia gravis. Neuromuscul Disord 2001;11:208–216.

26. Trastek VF, Payne WS. Surgery of the thymus gland. In: Shields TW: General thoracic surgery, 4th edn. Baltimore: Williams & Wilkins, 1994, pp 1124–1136.

27. Tsuchida M, Yamato Y, Souma T, et al. Efficacy and safety of extended thymectomy for elderly patients with myasthenia gravis. Ann Thorac Surg 1999;67:1563–1567.

28. Budde JM, Morris CD, Gal AA, Mansour KA, Miller JI. Predictors of outcome in thymectomy for myasthenia gravis. Ann Thorac Surg 2001;72:197–202.

29. Mulder DG. Extended transsternal thymectomy. Chest Surg Clin N Am 1996;6:95–105.

30. Pego-Fernandes P, Milanez de Campos J, Jatene F, Marchiori P, Suso F, Almeida de Oliveira S. Thymectomy by partial sternotomy for the treatment of myasthenia gravis. Ann Thorac Surg 2002;74:204–208.

31. Grandjean JG, Marco Lucchi M, Mariani MA. Reversed-T upper mini-sternotomy for extended thymectomy in myasthenic patients. Ann Thorac Surg 2000;70:1423–1424.

32. Masaoka A, Monden Y. Comparison of the results of transsternal simple, transcervical simple and extended thymectomy. Ann NY Acad Sci 1981;377:755–765.

33. Trastek VF. Thymectomy. In: Kaiser LR, Kron IL, Spray TL: Mastery of Cardiothoracic Surgery. Lippincott-Raven Eds, Philadelphia, 1998, pp 106.

34. Heiser JC, Rutherford RB, Ringel SP. Thymectomy for myasthenia gravis: a changing perspective. Arch Surg 1982;117:533–537.

35. Ciesla DJ, Moore EE, Woolford HY. Transverse sternal approach for thymectomy. Surgery 2003;133:226–227.

36. Venuta F, Rendina EA, De Giacomo T, et al. Thymectomy for myasthenia gravis: a 27-year experience. Eur J Cardiothorac Surg 1999;15:621–624.

37. Schumacher ED, Roth J. Thymektomie bei cenem Fall von Morbus Basedowii mit Myasthenie, Mit a. d. Grezgeb d. Med Chir 1912;25:746.

38. Kirschner PA, Osserman KE, Kark AE. Studies in myasthenia gravis: transcervical total thymectomy. JAMA 1969;209:906.

39. Cooper JD, Al-Jilaihawa AN, Pearson FG, Humphrey JG, Humphrey HE. An improved technique to facilitate transcervical thymectomy for myasthenia gravis. Ann Thorac Surg 1988;45:242–247.

40. Deeb ME, Brinster CJ, Kucharzuk J, Shrager JB, Kaiser LR. Expanded indications for transcervical thymectomy in the management of anterior mediastinal masses. Ann Thorac Surg 2001;72:208–211.

41. Kark AE, Kirschner PA. Total thymectomy by the transcervical approach. Br J Surg 1971;58:321–326.

42. Papatestas AE, Pozner J, Genkins G, Kornfeld P, Matta RJ. Prognosis in occult thymomas in myasthenia gravis following transcervical thymectomy. Arch Surg 1987;122:1352–1356.

43. Kojic J, Ilse WK, Cooper JD. Long-term clinical outcome after transcervical thymectomy for myasthenia gravis. Ann Thorac Surg 1998;65:1520–1522.

44. Calhoun RF, Ritter JH, Guthrie TJ, et al. Results of transcervical thymectomy for myasthenia gravis in 100 consecutive patients. Ann Surg 1999;230:555–559.

45. Ashour M. Prevalence of ectopic thymic tissue in myasthenia gravis and its clinical significance. J Thorac Cardiovasc Surg 1995;109:632–635.

46. Rossemberg M, Jaregui WO, DeVega ME, Errera MR, Roncoroni AJ. Recurrence of thymic hyperplasia after thymectmy in myasthenia gravis. Am J Med 1983;74:78–82.

47. Masaoka A, Monden Y, Seike Y, Tanioka T, Kagotani K. Reoperation after transcervical thymectomy for myasthenia gravis. Neurology 1982;32:83–85.

48. Jaretzki A III, Penn AS, Younger DS, et al. "Maximal" thymectomy for myasthenia gravis: results. J Thorac Cardiovasc Surg 1988;95:747–757.

49. Jaretzki A III. Transcervical/transsternal "maximal" thymectomy for myasthenia gravis. In: Shields T, LoCicero J, Ponn R, Eds. General thoracic surgery, 5th Ed. Lippincott Williams & Wilkins, Philadelphia, PA, 2000:2223–2232.

50. Jaretzki A III, Wolff M. "Maximal" thymectomy for myasthenia gravis. Surgical anatomy and operative technique. J Thorac Cardiovasc Surg 1988;96:711–716.

51. Jaretzki A III. Transcervical transsternal maximal thymectomy for myasthenia gravis (video), 1996. Soc Thorac Surg Libr, PO Box 809285, Chicago, IL, 60680–9285.

52. Sugarbaker DJ. Thoracoscopy in the management of anterior mediastinal masses. Ann Thorac Surg 1993;56:653–656.

53. Mack MJ. Video-assisted thoracic surgery. In Kaiser LR, Kron IL, Spray TL: Mastery of cardiothoracic surgery, Eds. Philadelphia: Lippincott-Raven, 1998, pp 92–104.

54. Rückert JC, Walter M, Müller JM. Pulmonary function after thoracoscopic thymectomy versus median sternotomy for myasthenia gravis. Ann Thorac Surg 2000;70: 1656–1661.

55. Jaretzki A III. Thymectomy for myasthenia gravis: analysis of controversies regarding technique and results. Neurology 1997;48(Suppl 5):S52–S63.

56. Savcenko M, Wendt GK, Prince SL, Mack MJ. Video-assisted thymectomy for myasthenia gravis: an update of a single institution experience. Eur J Cardiothorac Surg 2002 :22 :978–983.

57. Scelsi R, Ferro MT, Scelsi L, et al. Detection and morphology of thymic remnants after video-assisted thoracoscopic extended thymectomy (VATET) in patients with myasthenia gravis. Int Surg 1996;81:14–17.

58. Mineo TC, Pompeo E, Lerut TE, Bernardi G, Coosemans W, Nofroni I. Thoracoscopic thymectomy in autoimmune myasthenia: results of left-sided approach. Ann Thorac Surg 2000;69:1537–1541.

59. Yim APC, Kay RLC, Ho JKS. Video-assisted thoracoscopic thymectomy for myasthenia gravis. Chest 1995;108:1440–1443.

60. Novellino L, Longoni M, Spinelli L, et al. "Extended" thymectomy, without sternotomy, performed by cervicotomy and thoracoscopic technique in the treatment of myasthenia gravis. Int Surg 1994;79:378–381.

61. Mack MJ, Landreneau RJ, Yim AP, Hazelrigg SR, Scruggs GR. Results of video-assisted thymectomy in patients with myasthenia gravis. J Thorac Cardiovasc Surg 1996;112:1352–1359.

62. Yim AP. Thoracoscopic thymectomy: which side to approach? Ann Thorac Surg 1997;64:584–585.

63. Ruckert JC, Czyzewski D, Pest S, Muller JM. Radicality of thoracoscopic thymectomy – an anatomical study. Eur J Cardiothorac Surg 2000;18:735–736.

64. Mineo TC, Pompeo E, Ambrogi V. Video-assisted thoracoscopic thymectomy: from the right or from the left? J Thorac Cardiovasc Surg 1997;114:516–517.

65. Mineo TC, Pompeo E, Ambrogi V, et al. Adjuvant pneumomediastinum in thoracoscopic thymectomy for myasthenia gravis. Ann Thorac Surg 1996;62:1210–1212.

66. Granone P, Margaritora S, Cesario A, Galetta D. Thymectomy in myasthenia gravis via video-assisted inframammary cosmetic incision. Eur J Cardiothorac Surg 1999;15:861–863.

67. Yim APC, Izzat MB. VATS approach to the thymus. In Yim APC, et al. (eds): Minimal access cardiothoracic surgery. WB Saunders, Philadelphia, 2000.

68. Masaoka A, Yamakawa Y, Niwa H, et al. Extended thymectomy for myasthenia gravis patients: a 20-year review. Ann Thorac Surg 1996;62:853–859.

69. Frist WH, Thirumalai S, Doehring CB, et al. Thymectomy for the myasthenia gravis patient: factors influencing outcome. Ann Thorac Surg 1994;57:334–338.

70. Hatton PD, Diehl JT, Daly BD, et al. Transsternal radical thymectomy for myasthenia gravis: a 15-year review. Ann Thorac Surg 1989;47:838–840.

71. Matsuzaki Y, Tomita M, Onitsuka T, Shibata K. Influence of age on extended thymectomy as a treatment for myasthenia gravis. Ann Thorac Cardiovasc Surg 1998;4:192–195.

72. Nussbaum MS, Rosenthal GJ, Samaha FJ, Grinvalsky HT, Quinlan JG, Schmerler M, et al. Management of myasthenia gravis by extended thymectomy with anterior mediastinal dissection. Surgery 1992;112:681–688.

73. Olanow CW, Wechsler AS, Roses AD. A prospective study of thymectomy and serum acetylcholine receptor antibodies in myasthenia gravis. Ann Surg 1982;196:113–121.

74. Stern LE, Nussbaum MS, Quinlan JG, Fischer JE. Long-term evaluation of extended thymectomy with anterior mediastinal dissection for myasthenia gravis. Surgery 2001;130:774–778.

75. Roth T, Ackermann R, Stein R, Inderbitzi R, Rosler K, Schmid RA. Thirteen years follow-up after radical transsternal thymectomy for myasthenia gravis. Do short-term results predict long-term outcome? Eur J Cardiothorac Surg 2002;21:664–670.

76. Detterbeck FC, Scott WW, Howard JF Jr, et al. One hundred consecutive thymectomies for myasthenia gravis. Ann Thorac Surg 1996;62:242–245.

77. DeFilippi VJ, Richman DP, Ferguson MK. Transcervical thymectomy for myasthenia gravis. Ann Thorac Surg 1994;57:194–197.

78. Masaoka A, Monden Y, Seike Y, Tanioka T, Kagotani K. Reoperation after transcervical thymectomy for myasthenia gravis. Neurology 1982;32:83–85.

79. Jaretzki A 3rd, Penn AS, Younger DS, et al. "Maximal" thymectomy for myasthenia gravis. Results. J Thorac Cardiovasc Surg 1988;95:747–757.

80. Lennquist S, Andaker L, Lindvall B, Smeds S. Combined cervicothoracic approach in thymectomy for myasthenia gravis. Acta Chir Scand 1990;156:53–61.

81. Yim AP, Kay RL, Izzat MB, Ng SK. Video-assisted thoracoscopic thymectomy for myasthenia gravis. Semin Thorac Cardiovasc Surg 1999;11:65–73.

82. Mantegazza R, Baggi F, Bernasconi P, et al. Video-assisted thoracoscopic extended thymectomy and extended transsternal thymectomy (T-3b) in non-thymomatous myasthenia gravis patients: remission after 6 years of follow-up. J Neurol Sci 2003;212:31–36.

83. Gronseth GS, Barohn RJ. Practice parameter: thymectomy for autoimmune myasthenia gravis (an evidence-based review). Report of the Quality Standards Subcommittee of the American Academy of Neurology. Neurology 2000;55:7–15.

84. Kas J, Kiss D, Simon V, Svastics E, Major L, Szobor A. Decade-long experience with surgical therapy of myasthenia gravis: early complications of 324 transsternal thymectomies. Ann Thorac Surg 2001;72:1691–1697.

85. Maggi G, Casadio C, Cavallo A, Cianci R, Molinatti M, Ruffini E. Thymectomy in myasthenia gravis. Results of 662 cases operated upon 15 years. Eur J Cardiothorac Surg 1989;3:504–509.

86. Klein M, Heidenreich F, Madjlessi F, Granetzny A, Dauben HP, Schulte HD. Early and late results after thymectomy in myasthenia gravis: a retrospective study [correction of analysis]. Thorac Cardiovasc Surg 1999;47:170–173.

87. Jaretzki A 3rd, Barohn RJ, Ernstoff RM, et al. Myasthenia gravis: recommendations for clinical research standards. Task Force of the Medical Scientific Advisory Board of the Myasthenia Gravis Foundation of America. Neurology 2000;55:16–23.

88. Machens A, Busch CH, Emskötter TH, Izbicki JR. Morbidity after transsternal thymectomy for myasthenia gravis: a changing perspective? Thorac Cardiovasc Surg 1998;46:37–40.

89. Hankins JR, Mayer RF, Satterfield JR, et al. Thymectomy for myasthenia gravis: 14-year experience. Ann Surg 1985;201:618–625.

90. Spath G, Brinkmann A, Huth CH, Wiethölter H. Complications and efficacy of transsternal thymectomy in myasthenia gravis. Thorac Cardiovasc Surg 1987;35:283–289.

91. Remes-Troche JM, Tellez-Zenteno JF, Estanol B, Garduno-Espinoza J, Garcia-Ramos G. Thymectomy in myasthenia gravis: response, complications, and associated conditions. Arch Med Res 2002;33:545–551.

92. Jaretzki A III. Thymectomy for myasthenia gravis: analysis of controversies – patient management. The Neurologist 2003;9:77–92.

93. Fischer JE, Grinvalski HT, Nussbaum MS, Sayers HJ, Cole RE, Samaha FJ. Aggressive surgical approach for drug-free remission from myasthenia gravis. Ann Surg 1987;205:496–503.

94. Gracey DR, Divertie MB, Howard FM Jr, Payne WS. Postoperative respiratory care after transsternal thymectomy in myasthenia gravis. A 3-year experience in 53 patients. Chest 1984;86:67–71.

95. Younger DS, Braun NMT, Jaretzki A III, Penn AS, Lovelace RE. Myasthenia gravis: determinants for independent ventilation after transsternal thymectomy. Neurology 1984;34:336–340.

96. Naguib M, El Dawlatly AA, Ashour M, Bamgboye EA. Multivariate determinants of the need for postoperative ventilation in myasthenia gravis. Can J Anaesth 1996;43:1006–1013.

97. Cohn HE, Solit RW, Schatz NJ, Schlezinger N. Surgical treatment in myasthenia gravis. A 27 year experience. J Thorac Cardiovasc Surg 1974;68:876–885.

98. Molnar J, Szobor A. Myasthenia gravis: effect of thymectomy in 424 patients. A 15-year experience. Eur J Cardiothorac Surg 1990;4:8–14.

99. Durelli L, Maggi G, Casadio C, Ferri R, Rendine S, Bergamini L. Actuarial analysis of the occurrence of remissions following thymectomy for myasthenia gravis in 400 patients. J Neurosurg Psychiatry 1991;54:406–411.

100. Oosterhuis HJ. The natural course of myasthenia gravis: a long term follow up study. J Neurol Neurosurg Psychiatry 1989;52:1121–1127.

101. Klein M, Granetzny A, Dauben HP, Schulte HD, Gams E. Early and late results after thymectomy in myasthenia gravis: a retrospective analysis. Thorac Cardiovasc Surg 1999;47:170–173.

102. Nicolaou S, Muller NL, Li DK, Oger JJ. Thymus in myasthenia gravis: comparison of CT and pathologic findings and clinical outcome after thymectomy. Radiology 1996;201:471–474.

103. Cosi V, Romani A, Lombardi M, et al. Prognosis of myasthenia: a retrospective study of 380 patients. J Neurol 1997;244:548–555.

104. Bril V, Kojic J, Dhanani A. The long-term clinical outcome of myasthenia gravis in patients with thymoma. Neurology 1998;51:1198–1200.

105. de Perrot M, Liu J, Bril V, McRae K, Bezjak A, Keshavjee SH. Prognostic significance of thymomas in patients with myasthenia gravis. Ann Thorac Surg 2002;74:1658–1662.

106. Papatestas AE, Alpert LI, Osserman KE, Osserman RS, Kark AE. Studies in myasthenia gravis: effects of thymectomy. Results on 185 patients with nonthymomatous and thymomatous myasthenia gravis, 1941–1969. Am J Med 1971;50:465–474.

107. Monden Y, Nakahara K, Kagotani K, et al. Effects of preoperative duration of symptoms on patients with myasthenia gravis. Ann Thorac Surg 1984;38:287–291.

108. Matsushima S, Yamamoto H, Egami K, Suzuki S, Tanaka S. Evaluation of the prognostic factors after thymoma resection. Int Surg 2001;86:103–106.

109. Nakamura H, Taniguchi Y, Suzuki Y. Delayed remission after thymectomy for myasthenia gravis of the purely ocular type. J Thorac Cardiovasc Surg 1996;112:371–375.

110. Muller-Hermelink HK, Marx A. Pathological aspects of malignant and benign thymic disorders. Ann Med 1999;31(Suppl):5–14.

111. Perlo WP, Arnason B, Casterman B. The thymus gland in elderly patients with myasthenia gravis. Neurolgy 1975;25:294–295.

112. Donaldson DH, Ansher M, Horan S, Rutherford RB, Ringel SP. The relationship of age to outcome in myasthenia gravis. Neurology 1990;40:786–790.

113. Beghi E, Antozzi C, Batocchi AP, et al. Prognosis of myasthenia gravis: a multicenter follow-up study of 844 patients. J Neurol Sci 1991;106:213–220.

114. Monden Y, Nakahara K, Fujii Y, et al. Myasthenia gravis in elderly patients. Ann Thorac Surg 1985;39:433–436.

115. Tellez-Zenteno JF, Remes-Troche JM, Garcia-Ramos G, Estanol B, Garduno-Espinoza J. Prognostic factors of thymectomy in patients with myasthenia gravis: a cohort of 132 patients. Eur Neurol 2001;46:171–177.

116. Andrews PI, Massey JM, Howard JF Jr, Sanders DB. Race, sex, and puberty influence onset, severity, and outcome in juvenile myasthenia gravis. Neurology 1994;44:1208–1214.

117. Lindner A, Schalke B, Toyka KV. Outcome in juvenile-onset myasthenia gravis: a retrospective study with long-term follow-up of 79 patients. J Neurol 1997;244:515–520.

118. Adams C, Theodorescu D, Murphy EG, Shandling B. Thymectomy in juvenile myasthenia gravis. J Child Neurol 1990;5:215–218.

119. Kogut KA, Bufo AJ, Rothenberg SS, Lobe TE. Thoracoscopic thymectomy for myasthenia gravis in children. J Pediatr Surg 2000;35:1576–1577.

120. Kolski HK, Kim PC, Vajsar J. Video-assisted thoracoscopic thymectomy in juvenile myasthenia gravis. J Child Neurol 2001;16:569–573.

121. de Perrot M, Licker M, Spiliopoulos A. Factors influencing improvement and remission rates after thymectomy for myasthenia gravis. Respiration 2001;68:601–605.

122. Abt PL, Patel HJ, Marsh A, Schwartz SI. Analysis of thymectomy for myasthenia gravis in older patients: a 20-year single institution experience. J Am Coll Surg 2001;192:459–464.

123. Blossom GB, Ernstoff RM, Howells GA, Bendick PJ, Glover JL. Thymectomy for myasthenia gravis. Arch Surg 1993;128:855–862.

124. Busch C, Machens A, Pichlmeier U, Emskotter T, Izbicki JR. Long-term outcome and quality of life after thymectomy for myasthenia gravis. Ann Surg 1996;224:225–232.

125. Mantegazza R, Beghi E, Pareyson D, et al. A multicentre follow-up study of 1152 patients with myasthenia gravis in Italy. J Neurol 1990;237:339–344.

126. Lindstrom JM, Seybold ME, Lennon VA, et al. Antibody to acetylcholine receptor in myasthenia gravis: prevalence, clinical correlates and diagnostic value. Neurology 1976;26:1054–1059.

127. Mineo TC, Pompeo E, Ambrogi V, Bernardi G, Iani C, Sabato AF. Video-assisted completion thymectomy in refractory myasthenia gravis. J Thorac Cardiovasc Surg 1998;115:252–254.

128. Pompeo E, Nofroni I, Iavicoli N, Mineo TC. Thoracoscopic completion thymectomy in refractory nonthymomatous myasthenia. Ann Thorac Surg 2000;70:918–923.

129. Husain F, Ryan NJ, Hogan GR, Gonzalez E. Occurrence of invasive thymoma after thymectomy for myasthenia gravis: report of a case. Neurology 1990;40:170–171.

130. Hirabayashi H, Ohta M, Okumura M, Matsuda H. Appearance of thymoma 15 years after extended thymectomy for myasthenia gravis without thymoma. Eur J Cardiothorac Surg 2002;22:479–481.

131. Kirschner PA. Reoperation on the thymus. A Critique. Chest Surg Clin North Am 2001;11:439–445.

132. Henze A, Biberfeld P, Christensson B, Matell G, Pirskanen R. Failing transcervical thymectomy in myasthenia gravis. Scand J Thorac Cardiovasc Surg 1984;18:235–238.

133. Miller RG, Filler-Katz A, Kiprov D, Roan R. Repeat thymectomy in chronic refractory myasthenia gravis. Neurology 1991;41:923–924.

134. Graeber GM, Tamim W. Current status of the diagnosis and treatment of thymoma. Semin Thorac Cardiovasc Surg 2000;12:268–277.

135. Thomas CR, Wright CD, Loehrer PJ. Thymoma: state of the art. J Clin Oncol 1999;17:2280–2289.

136. Lara PN Jr. Malignant thymoma: current status and future directions. Cancer Treat Rev 2000;26:127–131.

137. Blumberg D, Port JL, Weksler B, et al. Thymoma: a multivariate analysis of factors predicting survival. Ann Thorac Surg 1995;60:908–913.

138. Loehrer PJ. Current approaches to the treatment of thymoma. Ann Med 1999;31(Suppl):73–79.

139. Rios A, Torres J, Galino PJ, et al. Prognostic factors in thymic epithelial neoplasms. Eur J Cardiothorac Surg 2002;21:307–313.

140. Myojin M, Choi NC, Wright CD, et al. Stage III thymoma: patern of failure after surgery and postoperative radiotherapy and its implication for future study. Int J radiat Oncol Biol Phys 2000;46:927–933.

141. Regnard JF, Magdeleinat P, Dromer C, et al. Prognostic factors and long-term results after thymoma resection: a series of 307 patients. J Thorac Cardiovasc Surg 1996;112:376–384.

142. Ogawa K, Uno T, Toita T, et al. Postoperative radiotherapy for patients with completely resected thymoma: a multi-institutional, retrospective review of 103 patients. Cancer 2002;94:1405–1413.

143. Wilkins KB, Sheikh E, Green R, et al. Clinical and pathologic predictors of survival in patients with thymoma. Ann Surg 1999;230:562–574.

144. Lewis JE, Wick MR, Scheithauer BW, Bernatz PE, Taylor WF. Thymoma. A clinicopathologic review. Cancer 1987;60:2727–4273.

145. Okumura M, Miyoshi S, Takeuchi, et al. Results of surgical treatment of thymoma with special reference to the invoved organs. J Thorac Cardiovasc Surg 1999;117:605–613.

146. Wang LS, Huang MH, Lin TS, Huang BS, Chien KY. Malignant thymoma. Cancer 1992;70:443–450.

147. Masaoka A, Monden Y, Nakahara K, Tanioka T. Follow-up study of thymoma with special reference to their clinical stages. Cancer 1981;48:2485–2492.

148. Matsushima S, Yamamoto H, Egami K, Suzuki S, Tanaka S. Evaluation of the prognostic factors after thymoma resection. Int Surg 2001;86:103–106.

149. Pescarmona E, Rendina EA, Venuta F, et al. Analysis of prognostic factors and clinicopathologic staging of thymoma. Ann Thorac Surg 1990;50:534–538.

150. Verley JM, Hollman KH. Thymoma. A comparative study of clinical stages, histologic features and survival in 200 cases. Cancer 1985;55:1074–1086.

151. Quintanilla-Martinez L, Wilkins EW Jr, Choi N, Efird J, Hug E, Harris NL. Thymoma: histologic subclassification is an independent prognostic factor. Cancer 1994;74:606–617.

152. Batata MA, Martini N, Huvos AG, Aguilar RI, Beattie EJ Jr. Thymomas: clinicopathologic features, therapy, and prognosis. Cancer 1974;34:389–396.

153. Wilkins EW Jr, Grillo HC, Scannell JG, Moncure AC, Mathisen DJ. J. Maxwell Chamberlain Memorial Paper. Role of staging in prognosis and management of thymoma. Ann Thorac Surg 1991;51:888–892.

154. Crucitti F, Doglietto GB, Bellantone R, et al. Effects of surgical treatment in thymoma with myasthenia gravis: our experience in 103 patients. J Surg Oncol 1992;50:43–46.

155. Etienne T, Deleaval PJ, Spiliopoulos A, Megevand R. Thymoma: prognostic factors. Eur J Cardiothorac Surg 1993;7:449–452.

156. Kohman LJ. Controversies in the management of malignant thymoma. Chest 1997;112(Suppl):S296–S300.

157. Lopez-Cano M, Ponseti-Bosch JM, Espin-Basany E, Sanchez-Garcia JL, Armengol-Carrasco M. Clinical and pathologic predictors of outcome in thymoma-associated myasthenia gravis. Ann Thorac Surg 2003;76:1643–1649.

158. Masaoka A, Yamakawa Y, Niwa H, et al. Thymectomy and malignancy. Eur J Cardiothorac Surg 1994;8:251–253.

159. Ruffini E, Mancuso M, Oliaro A, et al. Recurrence of thymoma: analysis of clinicopathologic features, treatment and outcome. J Thorac Cardiovasc Surg 1997;113:55–63.

160. Nakahara K, Ohno K, Hashimoto J, et al. Thymoma: results with complete resection and adjuvant postoperative irradiation in 141 consecutive patients. J Thorac Cardiovasc Surg 1988;95:1041–1047.

161. Monden Y, Nakahara K, Iioka S, et al. Recurrence of thymoma: clinicopathological features, therapy, and prognosis. Ann Thorac Surg 1985;39:165–169.

162. Haniuda M, Kondo R, Numanami H, Makiuchi A, Machida E, Amano J. Recurrence of thymoma: a clinicopathological feature, re-operation, and outcome. J Surg Oncol 2001;78:183–188.

163. Regnard JF, Zinzindohoue F, Magdeleinat P, Guibert L, Spaggiari L, Levasseur P. Results of Re-resection for Recurrent Thymomas. Ann Thorac Surg 1997;64:1593–1598.

164. Kirschner PA. Reoperation for thymoma: report of 23 cases. Ann Thorac Surg 1990;49:550–555.

165. Kattach H, Anastasiadis K, Cleuziou J, et al. Trans-sternal thymectomy for myasthenia gravis; surgical outcome. Ann Thorac Surg 2006;81:305–308.

Perioperative Management for Thymectomy

10

David Shlugman

Introduction

Myasthenia gravis (MG) is an autoimmune disease characterised by the production of auto-antibodies to the acetylcholine receptors on the post-junctional membrane of the neuromuscular junction. The reduction in the number of functional receptors gives rise to the cardinal feature of the disease: fatiguable weakness of the voluntary muscles. While playing a part in the disease process, the exact role of the thymus gland is unknown, as acetylcholine receptor (AChR) antibodies are produced here and in the periphery. However, thymectomy is associated with a fall in anti-acetylcholine receptor antibodies and an improvement in symptoms in most patients.

In the past, many anaesthetists avoided the use of muscle relaxants and routinely ventilated patients post operatively. However, with better understanding of the pathophysiology of the disease, and the advances in treatment, there has been a significant improvement in the morbidity and mortality of myasthenic patients undergoing thymic and non-thymic surgery.

Access to the thymus can be achieved by a number of surgical techniques, which are discussed elsewhere. These include the transsternal and transcervical approaches and, in recent years, the minimally invasive video-assisted thoracoscopic approach. As the transsternal approach is the only one used in this institution, discussion will relate to this surgical technique, although the principles involved in anaesthetising a patient with MG will remain the same.

Assessment

Pre-operative assessment of the myasthenic patient aims to:
1. Establish the severity of the disease
2. Review the course of the disease in the past, including crises and admissions to hospital
3. Review confirmatory evidence from the special investigations
4. Review the treatment regimen
5. Establish the presence or absence of a thymic tumour
6. Review fitness for thoracic surgery
7. Establish co-morbid conditions

Classification of Myasthenia Gravis

Osserman and Genkins published a classification of the various stages of the disease in 1971 [1]. In 2001, Baraka published a simplified and modified version which is more practical and can be used as a predictor of post-operative complications [2].

0. Asymptomatic
1. Ocular signs and symptoms only
2. Generalised mild muscle weakness only
3. Generalised moderate weakness or bulbar dysfunction
4. Acute fulminating presentation or respiratory dysfunction
5. Late severe generalised myasthenia gravis

Clinical Features and Diagnosis

Most patients will present with ocular signs (ptosis, diplopia), with other manifestations (bulbar, limb, respiratory muscles) usually becoming evident within three years of initial presentation. It is a disease marked by remissions and exacerbations, the latter precipitated by infection (especially respiratory and gastro-intestinal), stress, overtreatment, pregnancy, low serum potassium, and drugs (aminoglycoside antibiotics, tetracyclines, β-blockers). Neck and proximal muscle groups are most commonly affected. Bulbar dysfunction is characterised by difficulty with chewing and swallowing, and speech is usually nasal in quality. Nasal regurgitation and pulmonary aspiration are not uncommon. An inability to take a deep breath and cough effectively is indicative of diaphragmatic involvement. An anti-AChR antibody assay will confirm the diagnosis, although up to 20% of myasthenics are seronegative for the antibody. There is no correlation between the antibody titre and severity of disease. Besides other confirmatory tests for MG (edrophonium test, neurophysiological studies), a chest

X-ray is important to exclude a thymic tumour. If found, a CT scan or MRI will indicate its size and may reveal its attachment to adjacent structures, e.g. pericardium, great vessels and pleura. Proximity to or involvement of the tumour with the phrenic nerve(s) will influence the post-operative management significantly.

Treatment

Treatment aims to:
1. Enhance neuromuscular transmission with anticholinesterase agents
2. Decrease antibody production via immunosuppressants (azathioprine, cyclosporine A), steroid therapy and thymectomy
3. Temporarily decreasing circulating antibodies or plasmapharesis with intravenous immunoglobulins

Pyridostigmine, rather than neostigmine, is the anticholinesterase of choice. It has a slower onset of action (30–60 min), but a longer duration of action (3–4 h) necessitating its use up to five times a day in severe cases. It is available as an oral preparation, and its side effects of colic, increased salivation and sweating can be unpleasant. Debate arises as to whether pyridostigmine should be omitted on the day of surgery because of its antagonistic effect on muscle relaxants and the increase in bronchial secretions. A pragmatic approach is to assess the severity of the myasthenia, both subjectively and objectively. Generally speaking, patients with the milder form of the disease (ocular involvement) are able to omit the pre-operative dose of the drug. High dose anti-cholinesterase and steroid therapy, repeated hospital admissions, frequent need for plasma exchanges and immunoglobulin therapy, however, are suggestive of severe disease. Many patients are also psychologically dependent on pyridostigmine. In these cases, it is better to allow the patient to take the drug on the day of surgery. In practice, this does not seem to have an adverse effect on the conduct of the anaesthetic besides an increased requirement for muscle relaxants.

Steroid therapy needs to be continued and augmented during the perioperative period. Immunosupressants are avoided on the day of surgery because of their potential effect on the empty stomach. A full blood count, clotting tests and a random blood glucose are done and two units of blood cross. Pre-medication is with an H_2 antagonist and metoclopramide. Potentially respiratory depressant drugs, e.g. benzodiazepines, are avoided.

Examination

Examination aims to:
1. Assess the patient's fitness for thoracic surgery
2. Exclude autoimmune disorders associated with myasthenia gravis (thyroid disease, rheumatoid arthritis, systemic)

Fortuitously is an anterior mediastinal structure lying immediately posterior to the sternum. Except for thymomas, which invade adjacent structures, dissection of the gland from surrounding tissues is relatively simple and quickly achieved. As most patients presenting for thoracotomy are usually under 50 years of age, significant co-morbidities are not common. It is essential to optimise the patient's condition prior to surgery, even if this requires cancellation of the operation to allow for drug regimen manipulation, plasmapharesis or immunoglobulin therapy. It has been shown that patients who underwent plasmapheresis before thymectomy required less post-operative ventilation (1 day vs. 2.7 days) and had a shorter stay in the intensive care unit (3.1 days vs. 4.5 days) [3].

Assessment

Discussion with the patient as part of informed consent should stress the absolute necessity for an ICU/HDU bed post-operatively, the lack of which would preclude surgery. Occasionally a blood transfusion may be required, usually associated with resection of an invasive thymic tumour while, in rare instances, post-operative ventilation in the ICU may be necessary. It is also important to stress the lack of severe post-operative pain. Recovery and discharge from hospital is quick, with uncomplicated cases usually leaving hospital within a week following surgery.

With the current shortage of ICU and HDU beds in the UK, a decision should be made as to the destination of patient immediately post operatively as this could make the difference to whether the operation will proceed or not. It is possible to predict those who may require elective post-operative ventilation. Four risk factors were indentified by Leventhal et al [4] in 1980:
1. duration of MG > 6 years
2. presence of coexisting respiratory disease
3. pyridostigmine dose > 750 mg/day
4. vital capacity < 2.9 litres.

However, the improvement in treatment options over the last quarter of a century (steroid therapy, plasmapharesis, immunoglobulin therapy) has resulted in today's patient presenting for surgery in far better condition than previously, thus reducing the number requiring elective post-operative ventilation [5]. Broadly speaking, those patient with brittle disease, on high doses of anti-cholinesterases, and who have been admitted to hospital on numerous occasions for exacerbations of disease, are most likely to be problematic.

Anaesthetic Management

Techniques

The anaesthetic techniques fall into 3 groups:
1. muscle relaxant or non-muscle relaxant technique
2. inhalational versus intravenous route
3. regional blockade with light general anaesthesia

Muscle Relaxants

The response of myasthenics to depolarizing and non-depolarising (competitive) muscle relaxants can be variable and is dependent on the severity of the disease and the patient's treatment regimen. It is thought the paucity of post-synaptic acetylcholine receptors or their functional blockade by anti-AChR antibodies accounts for the so-called resistance to suxamethonium, as the drug has fewer binding sites. The effect clinically is a partial or inadequate neuromuscular block to a standard dose. To achieve satisfactory intubating conditions for a rapid sequence technique, a dose of 1.5–2 mg/kg suxamethonium is recommended [6]. The neuromuscular response is complicated, however, by the plasma cholinesterase activity, which is reduced by the anticholinesterase treatment. Consequently, there can be a prolongation in the duration of a depolarizing block in patients on anticholinesterase treatment, especially if the anticholinesterase was taken immediately prior to surgery [7]. Those patients in true remission from the disease, and off all anticholinesterase therapy, demonstrate a normal response to suxamethonium [8]. Mivacurium is the only competitive muscle relaxant that is hydrolysed to inactive metabolites by plasma cholinesterase. Use of this drug in myasthenics illustrates the need for a significantly reduced dosage of competitive muscle relaxants to achieve a desired effect. Like suxamethonium, there is a prolongation of action of mivacurium as a result of reduced circulating plasma cholinesterase levels [9, 10].

The competitive muscle relaxants atracurium and vecuronium have safely been used in myasthenic patients since the 1980s. Myasthenics require 1/10th the dose necessary for a normal patient. Atracurium undergoes spontaneous decomposition (Hoffman elimination) and ester hydrolysis, which is independent of plasma cholinesterase, resulting in a lack of cumulative effect. This makes it ideally suited for use in myasthenic patients. An initial intubating dose of 0.1–0.2 mg/kg will provide a 30–40 min duration of effect with incremental doses of 1 mg prolonging the block by 10 to 20 min [11, 12]. For vecuronium, the intubating dose is 10–40 mcg/kg with incremental doses of 4–5 mcg/kg every 22 min [13, 14]. With vecuronium, it has been shown the greater the anti-AChR antibodies titre, the more sensitive the my-

asthenic patient is to the drug [15]. Patients with only ocular symptoms require higher doses of vecuronium compared to those patients with generalised symptoms, with the onset of block taking longer in the former group [16]. Rocuronium has also been used satisfactorily in a myasthenic patient undergoing transsternal thymectomy, and displayed similar properties to atracurium and vecuronium [17]. Long-acting relaxants like pancuronium are considered unsuitable [18].

Most anaesthetists accept adequate recovery of neuromuscular function with a TOF >0.70. An interesting study by Eriksson et al. [19] demonstrated that in spite of an adductor pollicis TOF ratio ≥0.70 following the administration of vecuronium to awake normal subjects, half still showed pharyngeal dysfunction. Pharyngeal function only normalised with a TOF >0.90. Another study [20] in healthy awake volunteers found a TOF >0.70–0.75 was associated with diplopia, decreased grip strength and an inability to sit up, but yet an ability to perform a 5 sec. head-lift. Even a TOF >0.85–0.90 was associated with visual symptoms and generalised fatigue. Although similar studies have not been done in myasthenic patients, it is conceivable that this group of patients would be particularly susceptible to the effects of an inadequate reversal of the muscle relaxants, in spite of an "adequate" TOF >0.70.

In summary, depolarizing and short-acting competitive muscle relaxants can be used with safety in myasthenic patients, so long as the dose is titrated to effect and some form of monitoring of neuromuscular function is used.

Epidural Anaesthesia

A non-muscle relaxant technique in conjunction with epidural anaesthesia is a useful, albeit more complicated alternative [21]. It also provides excellent post-operative analgesia in a group of patients whose ability to cough and clear secretions may not be optimal [22, 23].

Inhalational Agents

All inhalational agents depress neuromuscular transmission, with the effect being more profound in myasthenic patients [24]. A number of mechanisms are involved, including the inhibition of presynaptic acetylcholine and its mobilization and release, and effects on the post-junctional membrane [25, 26]. It is dose- and agent-dependent. Clinically, it manifests as a prolongation of action of the competitive muscle relaxants, with a consequent diminished requirement for these agents. Sevoflurane prolonged the neuromuscular block maximally, followed by enflurane, isoflurane and halothane [26].

Intravenous Agents

A total intravenous technique with propofol does not affect neuromuscular function [27] and has the added advantage of ease of titratability, rapid recovery and an anti-emetic effect.

Thus, it would seem all anaesthetic techniques are suitable for the myasthenic patient, with the choice ultimately being operator-dependent. In the light of the above, however, it may be preferable to use intravenous agents without muscle relaxants for the severe myasthenic patient.

Current Technique at Oxford

The following is a description of the technique used by the author for the trans-sternal approach. Prior to the arrival of the patient in the anaesthetic room, the availability of an ICU/HDU bed is confirmed, as well as the presence of two units of cross matched blood in the operating theatre refrigerator. The defibriletor, internat paddles and connections are checked and placed in the operating theatre ready for immediate use in the event of ventricular fibrillation occuring.

Anaesthesia

On arrival in the anaesthetic room, an anxiolytic dose of intravenous midazolam is given. While the patient breaths oxygen via a face mask, a peripheral nerve stimulator is placed over the posterior tibial nerve. Using TCI propofol, anaesthesia is induced and maintained, and the patient allowed to breathe spontaneously on nitrous oxide and oxygen via a face mask. If required, the ventilation may be assisted manually. A baseline train of four stimuli (2 Hz every 10 sec) is acquired, following which atracurium 10 mg is given. A full 3 min. is allowed to elapse before the TOF is tested again. If a twitch is still present a further 10 mg atracurium is given. This sequence is repeated until there is total abolition of motor function of the toes to further stimulation. Neuromuscular transmission is monitored throughout the surgery. Fentanyl is given, followed by oral tracheal intubation with a reinforced tracheal tube. An arterial line and a 14 g intravenous cannula are sited on the same arm, and the patient moved into the operating theatre. Central venous and urinary catheters have been found not to be necessary. A prophylactic antibiotic is given. Aminoglycosides and polymyxins are avoided, as they are known to depress neuromuscular transmission [28].

Surgery

Prior to skin incision, the tissues overlying the sternum are infiltrated with 20 ml of bupivicaine 0.5% and a further dose of fentanyl is given to obtund the pressor response to sternotomy. Amide (bupivicaine), as opposed to ester local anaesthetics (procaine, tetracaine), are preferable as they usually does not exacerbate the symptoms of myasthenia. An exacerbation has been reported following the use of the amide local anaesthetic mepivicaine for an axillary block [2]. Immediately prior to sternotomy, the patient is disconnected from the ventilator to prevent damage to the underlying lung and pleura. Thymectomy (for non-thymoma surgery) is a relatively simple operation by virtue of the gland's location in the anterior mediastinum with minimal attachment to surrounding structures. Damage to the phrenic nerves must be avoided at all costs during the resection. An opening in the pleural cavity is not of major significance, so long as the visceral pleura remains intact. Should the latter be breached, an alveolar leak will result.

Because of the tumour's ability to infiltrate adjacent structures, a thymoma resection can transform a relatively simple operation into a major procedure. Tumour infiltration of the pericardium and major vessels, as well as extension into the recesses of the pleural cavity, can make this a hazardous procedure. From the CT scan, it is often possible to predict such problematic cases, and in these circumstances it may be wise to perform the surgery in centres where cardio-thoracic expertise and equipment are readily available. The phrenic nerve(s) are often enmeshed in the tumour mass, and damage to both should be avoided at all costs, as a bilateral nerve palsy in a myasthenic patient is disastrous.

After resection of the gland, haemostasis is achieved and the two halves of the sternum wired together. A mediastinal drain is left in situ, as are pleural drains should the parietal pleura have been breached. Blood loss is usually modest and blood transfusion an uncommon event.

Post-operative Care

For the last 10 years, all our patients have been extubated at the end of surgery. Prior to the administration of the reversal agent, the peripheral nerve stimulator is checked for return of motor function. Following extubation, the patient is transferred to the ICU/HDU for observation for a minimum of 24 h. A post-operative chest-x-ray is done to exclude a pneumothorax or haemothorax, and an attempt is made to assess the level of the diaphragms at this early stage. Blood loss from the drain sites needs to be monitored carefully, as it may the only sign of early bleeding in the young patient. Post-operative pain is readily controlled with a fentanyl infusion, oral analgesics and non-steroidal anti-inflammatories. Pyridostigmine is omitted for the first 24 h post-operatively and recommenced at half the usual dose on the second day. Full dosage is resumed by the third post-operative day. The reason for the lesser requirement immediately after surgery is unexplained.

References

1. Osserman KE, Genkins G. Studies in myasthenia gravis: review of a twenty-year experience in over 1200 patients. Mt Sinai J Med 1971;38:497–537.

2. Baraka A. Anesthesia and critical care of thymectomy for myasthenia gravis. Chest Surg Clin North Am 2001;11:337–361.

3. d'Empaire G, Hoaglin DC, Perlo VP, et al. Effect of pre-thymectomy plasma exchange on postoperative respiratory function in myasthenia gravis. J Thor Cardiovasc Surg 1985;89:592–596.

4. Leventhal SR, Orkin FK, Hirsh RA. Prediction of the need for postoperative mechanical ventilation in myasthenia gravis. Anaesth 1980;53:26–30.

5. Chevalley C, Spiliopoulos A, de Perrot M, et al. Perioperative medical management and outcome following thymectomy for myasthenia gravis. Can J Anaesth 2001;48:446–451.

6. Eisenkraft JB, Book WJ, Mann SM, et al. Resistance to succinylcholine in myasthenia gravis. Anaesth 1988;69:760–763.

7. Baraka A. Suxamethonium block in the myasthenic patient. Anaesth 1992;47:217–219.

8. Abel M, Eisenkraft JB, Patel N. Response to suxamethonium in a myasthenic patient during remission. Anaesth 1991;46:30–32.

9. Seigne RD, Scott RPF. Mivacurium chloride and myasthenia gravis. Br J Anaesth 1994;72:468–469.

10. Paterson IG, Hood JR, Russell SH, et al. Mivacurium in the myasthenic patient. Br J Anaesth 1994;73:494–498.

11. Baraka A, Dajani A. Atracurium in myasthenics undergoing thymectomy. Anesth Analg 1984;63:1127–1130.

12. Smith CE, Donati F, Bevan DR. Cumulative dose-response curves for atracurium in patients with myasthenia gravis. Can J Anaesth 1989;36:402–406.

13. Hunter JM, Bell CF, Florence AM, et al. Vecuronium in the myasthenic patient. Anaesth 1985;40:848–853.

14. Eisenkraft JB, Book WJ, Papatestas AE. Sensitivity to vecuronium in myasthenia gravis: a dose-response study. Can J Anaesth 1990;37:301–306.

15. Nillson E, Meretoja OA. Vecuronium dose-response and maintenance requirements in patients with myasthenia gravis. Anesth 1990;73:28–32.

16. Itoh H, Shibata K, Nitta S. Difference in sensitivity to vecuronium between patients with ocular and generalized myasthenia gravis. Br J Anaesth 2001;87:885–889.

17. Baraka A, Haroun-Bizri S, Kawas N, et al. Rocuronium in the myasthenic patient. Anaesth 1995;50:1007.

18. Kopman AF, Ng J, Zank LM, et al. Residual postoperative paralysis. Anaesth 1996;85:1253–1259.

19. Eriksson LI, Sundman E, Olsson R et al. Functional assessment of the pharynx at rest and during swallowing in partially paralyzed humans. Anaesth 1997;87:1035–1043.

20. Kopman AF, Yee PS, Neuman GG. Relationship of the train-of-four fade ratio to clinical signs and symptoms of residual paralysis in awake volunteers. Anaesth 1997;86:765–771.

21. Akpolat N, Tilgen H, Gursoy F, et al. Thoracic epidural and analgesia with bupivicaine for transsternal thymectomy for myasthenia gravis. Eur J Anaesth 1997;14:220–223.

22. El-Dawlatly AA, Ashour MH. Anaesthesia for thymectomy in myasthenia gravis. A non-muscle relaxant technique. Anaesth Intensive Care 1994;22:458–460.

23. Tortosa JA, Hernandez-Palazon J. Anaesthesia for laparoscopic cholecystectomy in myasthenia gravis: a non muscle relaxant technique. Anaesth 1997;52:807–808.

24. Abel M, Eisenkraft JB. Anesthetic implications of myasthenia gravis. Mt Sinai J Med 2002;69:31–37.

25. Nilsson E, Muller K. Neuromuscular effects of isoflurane in patients with myasthenia gravis. Acta Anaesth Scand 1990;34:126–131.

26. Saitoh Y, Toyooka H, Amaha K. Recoveries of post-tetanic twitch and train-of-four responses after administration of vecuronium with different inhalational anaesthetics and neurolept anaesthesia. Br J Anaesth 1993;70: 402–404.

27. O'Flaherty D, Pennant J, Rao K, et al. Total intravenous anaesthesia with propofol for transsternal thymectomy in myasthenia gravis. J Clin Anesth 1992;4:241–244.

28. Pittinger CB, Eryasa Y, Adamson R. Antibiotic-induced paralysis. Anesth Analg 1970; 49:487–501.

29. de Jose Maria B, Carrero E, Sala X. Myasthenia gravis and regional anaesthesia. Can J Anaesth 1995;42:178–179.

Systemic Treatment of Thymoma

11

Penny Bradbury and Denis Talbot

Background

Surgery is the treatment of choice for thymoma, with excellent cure rates in early stage disease. In the setting of more advanced thymoma, long-term survival is more difficult to achieve. This has resulted in the use of more complex multi-modality treatment protocols designed to downstage inoperable disease and to treat micro-metastases. It is in this setting that chemotherapy has an increasing role, in addition to its use in the palliative setting.

Thymoma is a chemosensitive malignancy, with responses documented to a range of drugs [1]. Due to the low prevalence of thymoma, evidence for efficacy of chemotherapy is restricted to case reports and phase II studies, with relatively small numbers of patients. It is, therefore, an evolving area requiring on-going research to define optimum treatment protocols. As with the study of other rare diseases, it is important that international and multi-centre co-operation is fostered. This chapter will discuss the evidence for systemic treatment of thymoma and the increasing role of chemotherapy in the multimodality treatment of the disease.

Single Agent Cisplatin

Of the many drugs that have been reported to have activity in thymoma, the greatest evidence exists for the use of cisplatin and corticosteroids. The first published report of the use of cisplatin in thymoma was in 1973 [2]. A single patient had a partial response (defined as a 50% reduction in the product of the perpendicular dimensions of the tumour [3]) when cisplatin was administered in a low dose, conducted as part of a phase I trial. Since then, there have been several reports documenting the efficacy of single agent cisplatin in advanced thymoma, with response rates varying between 11 and 100% in small series (reviewed by Hejna et al. [1]).

In retrospective study of 87 patients with thymoma treated at the M.D. Anderson Cancer Center between 1951 and 1990, 17 patients were treated with cisplatin alone or in combination with corticosteroids. In this series the response rate to single agent cisplatin was 64% [4]. A disappointing response rate to just 11% was reported in a series of 24 patients with recurrent or metastatic thymoma treated with cisplatin at a dose of 50 mg/m^2, leading the authors to conclude that single agent cisplatin was ineffective at this relatively low dose [5]. A later review of the literature [1] reported a response rate of 43% among trials that had used cisplatin with doses of up to 130 mg/m^2.

While response rates in some studies are impressive, there are no randomised trials comparing treatment with best supportive care in the advanced setting. Park et al. demonstrated a significantly longer median survival in patients who responded to chemotherapy compared with non-responders [4]. Patients who responded to chemotherapy had a median survival of 67 months, versus 17 months in those who did not, suggesting a potential survival benefit associated with chemotherapy [4].

Corticosteroids

There have been reports of the activity of corticosteroids and ACTH in the treatment of malignant thymoma since 1952 [6]. Regimens that have been used include prednisone (30–60 mg daily), ACTH (25 mg, four times per day) and dexamethasone (16 mg daily) as reviewed by Hu and Levine [7]. Remissions of up to three years have been reported in all histological subtypes [8]. Unfortunately, relapses frequently occur after cessation of treatment, although second remissions have been reported with the use of steroids to threat initial relapse [8].

It has been well documented that corticosteroids can reduce the lymphocyte population within the tumour, leading to a different epithelial predominant subtype. It has been an area of debate whether corticosteroids have a direct effect on the malignant epithelial cells or act merely to reduce the lymphocyte population. There is some evidence to suggest that corticosteroids may have an effect on the epithelial population within a thymoma. Glucocorticoid receptors are present within the epithelial cytoplasm of radiation-induced thymomas in mouse models [9]. A study of the histological changes in 14 patients treated with corticosteroids prior to surgery described the presence of epithelial cells, with pyknotic nuclei and eosinophilic cytoplasm similar to lympho-cytes, after exposure to corticosteroids in some cases. In addition, the apoptotic index of the epithelial cells was increased and the MIB-1, a marker of proliferation, in-dex was decreased [10]. Whether this represents a direct effect of steroids on epithelial cells, or involves a more complex interplay between lymphocytes and the epithe-lial component of the tumour, is unclear.

Thus, corticosteroids provide a useful treatment op-tion, particularly for patients with advanced disease and a performance status that precludes more aggressive treat-ment. It is not, however, without risk to the patient, as fungal infections secondary to the immunosuppressive effects of steroids have been frequently described in trials assessing the efficacy of steroids in thymoma [7, 10].

Other Single Agents

Other drugs that have been used in the treatment of thy-moma include ifosfamide, doxorubicin and the cytokine interleukin-2 (IL-2). In a trial of single agent ifosfamide among 13 patients with stage III or stage IVB disease, there were 5 complete and one partial response (46%), with an estimated 57% survival at 5 years [11].

Cytotoxic lymphocytes are activated in the presence of IL-2, providing a theoretical explanation of the mode of action of IL-2 in the treatment of some malignancies. A single case report described a rapid response to IL-2 in a heavily pre-treated patient with advanced thymoma, but unfortunately in a study of 14 patients there were no responses [12, 13]. Assessment of the efficacy of other drugs has been limited to small numbers of case reports, and their role is yet to be fully defined. Table 11.1 sum-marises the data for drugs reported to have activity as single agents in the treatment of thymoma.

Combination Chemotherapy

Combination chemotherapy is commonly used in the treatment of cancer. Typically, in the design of combina-tion regimens, drugs with different modes of action are chosen, thereby increasing response rates and exploiting synergy. A second consideration relates to the side effects of drugs. An ideal combination regimen has components with non-overlapping toxicities.

Combination chemotherapy has been shown to be superior to single agent treatment of thymoma, and on the basis of its activity as a single agent most regimens include cisplatin. The largest published study of patients with advanced thymoma treated with combination che-motherapy used a regimen now frequently referred to as ADOC. This regimen consists of cisplatin (50mg/m^2 on day 1), doxorubicin (40 mg/m^2 on day 1), vincristine (0.6 mg/m^2 on day 3) and cyclophosphamide (700mg/m^2 on day 4) repeated every 28 days [14]. Of 37 patients with stage III or IV thymoma five had previously been treated with surgery or radiotherapy or both; the remaining 32 patients had not received prior treatment. An overall re-sponse rate of 92% was reported, with a median survival of 15 months. ADOC has now become one of the most

Table 11.1 Single of agents with reported activity in thymoma

Drug	No. of patients	Dose/schedule	Response rate	CR	PR	Author/ [Ref]
Cisplatin	24	50 mg/m^2 3 times a week	2/20	–	2	Bonomi et al. [5]
	17*	Not available	11/17	6	5	Park et al. [4]
	1	As part of phase 1 trial	1/1	–	1	Talley et al. [2]
	1	120 mg/m^2 3 times a week	1/1	1	–	
Corticosteroids	1	ACTH 25 mg 4 times a day	1/1	–	1	Sofer L.F. [6]
	12	Review of 7 trials**	10/12	3	7	Hu and Levine [7]
Ifosfamide	15	1.5 g days 1–5	6/13	5	1	Highley et al. [11]
Doxorubicin	3	Not Available	2/3	–	2	Hu and Levine [7]
Interleukin 2	1	20 x 10(6) IU/m^2/day for 5 days x2	1	–	1	Berthaud et al. [12]
	14	12 x 10(6) IU/m^2/day for 5 days for 4 weeks	0/14	–	–	Gordon et al. [13]

* Some patients had concomitant corticosteroids. Adapted from Hu and Levine 1986 [7]
** Including prednisone 30 mg daily, 60 mg daily, or dexamethasone 16 mg daily

frequently used regimens in the treatment of thymoma [14].

Other chemotherapy combinations include cisplatin, doxorubicin and cyclophosphamide (PAC) and etoposide, ifosphamide and cisplatin(VIP). In a trial of 30 patients with advanced or relapsed thymoma or thymic carcinoma treated with PAC (cisplatin 50mg/m^2, doxorubicin 50mg/m^2 and cyclophosphamide 500mg/m^2 with treatment repeated every 21 days), an overall response rate of 50% was seen (3 complete and 12 partial responses) with a median survival of 38 months [15]. In a similar trial using VIP (etoposide 75m/m^2 on days 1-4, ifosfamide 1.2g/m^2 on days 1-4 and cisplatin 20mg/m^2 on days 1–4 with treatment repeated every 21 days) among 28 assessable patients with advanced thymoma or thymic carcinoma there were 9 partial responses and a median survival of 32 months. These results appeared inferior to those reported in other phase II trials [16]. More impressive results were reported in a phase II trial of cisplatin and etoposide (cisplatin 60mg/m^2 on day 1and etoposide 120mg/m^2 on days 1–3). Among 16 patients with recurrent or metastatic thymoma, 5 complete responses and 4 partial responses were described with a survival time of 4.3 years. These results appear similar to those achieved with PAC [17].

Toxicity can increase with combination chemotherapy, but most trials have reported an acceptable level of toxicity. For example, in the trial examining the efficacy of ADOC there were no grade IV toxicities. Grade III nausea and vomiting were the most common toxicities occurring in 70% of patients. Grade III leukopenia occurred in 22% of patients [14–17].

An interesting and less toxic approach has been to use the combination of the somatostatin analogue octreotide and prednisone. Approximately 30% of tumours take up octreotide as assessed by octreoscan. Of 38 patients with advanced thymoma or thymic carcinoma and positive octreoscans treated with octreotide and prednisone, there were 2 complete and 10 partial responses. On the balance of evidence, octreotide has activity in the advanced setting and is well tolerated, an important consideration when treatment is given with palliative intent [18]. This approach warrants further investigation.

Multi-Modality Treatment

With evidence to support the use of chemotherapy in patients with inoperable disease, it is now becoming a component of the multi-modality treatment of thymoma. Surgical resection of early stage disease provides the best chance of cure. Following relapse the disease becomes difficult to cure. Recurrent disease after resection indicates the presence of occult micro-metastasis that could potentially have been treated with systemic adjuvant therapy soon after surgery. The successful use of adjuvant treatment as standard treatment of early stage breast and colon cancer is supported by evidence in large randomised trials. The place of adjuvant chemotherapy in thymoma is less clear. In a retrospective study of 149 patients with thymoma, 74 (50%) had received chemotherapy and radiotherapy after surgery. Multivariate analysis indicated that the lack of chemotherapy was one of four characteristics that conferred a poorer prognosis [19]. Two other trials provide supportive evidence for the use of adjuvant therapy. A retrospective study of 200 patients treated at the Shanghai Chest Hospital showed that patients with WHO histological subtypes B2, B3 or C who had received adjuvant therapy had a better 5 year survival than those treated with surgery alone (85.5% vs. 48.3% log rank p=<0.002). Only eight of the patients within this group, however, received adjuvant chemotherapy. Thus, only limited conclusions can be drawn from these data [20]. A trial of post-operative chemotherapy in 13 patients, 8 with thymoma and 7 with thymic carcinoma, described a complete remission in 8 patients who had undergone partial surgical debulking. Relapse occurred in 7 patients, with a median time to recurrence of nine months (Milstein et al., reviewed in Hejna et al. [1]). Without randomised trials, however, the true benefit of adjuvant chemotherapy is unknown. Adjuvant chemotherapy is not part of current clinical practice.

Neo-adjuvant chemotherapy is the use of chemotherapy before definitive local treatment such as surgery. It is employed to down stage initially inoperable disease. Neo-adjuvant chemotherapy has potential advantages over adjuvant therapy or surgery alone. Pre-operative chemotherapy is generally better tolerated than post-operative treatment, allowing a high proportion of the planned dose (Dose Intensity) to be administered. It also has the potential to downstage the disease, improving the chance of surgical resection. Neo-adjuvant chemotherpay provides early treatment of micro-metastases. Despite these theoretical advantages there have been no randomised trials to assess the efficacy of this approach. Induction chemotherapy is supported by phase II data and is frequently used in the treatment of locally advanced disease. Regimens that have been assessed for neo-adjuvant therapy are those that were most efficacious in advanced disease, namely ADOC and PAC.

Table 11.2 summarises seven trials (six prospective) in which chemotherapy was incorporated into multi-modality protocols for advanced thymoma. The trials were heterogeneous, using different chemotherapy regimens and different radiotherapy protocols. Comparisons are, therefore, difficult to make. The overall response rates in trials using neo-adjuvant chemotherapy are high, ranging between 70% and 100%.

The largest study of patients comes from a review of six trials by Tomiak and Evans [21]. In that study, 61 patients with stage III or IV disease were given chemotherapy, of which 22 proceeded to surgery. Of these, 11 had com-

Table 11.2 Trials incorporating neo-adjuvant chemotherapy in the multimodality treatment of thymoma

Treatment	Stage	No. of patients	Chemotherapy	Complete resection	Response rate	Author [Ref]
C-S-R	III, IVA	61 (retrospective review of 6 trials)	49/61 cisplatin-based	11	89% 19 CR 35 PR	Tomiak and Evans [21]
C-S-R*	III, IVA	16	Cisplatin Cyclophosphamide Doxorubicin Vincristine	11	100% 7/16 CR 9/16 PR	Rea, Sartori et al. [22]
C-S-R	IIIA	7	Cisplatin Epirubicin Etoposide	4	100% 7 PR	Macchiarini, Chella et al. [34]
C-S-C	III, IVA	16	Cisplatin Cyclophosphamide Doxorubicin Vincristine	9	81% 2 11	Berruti, Borasio et al. [23]
C-S-R-C	III, IVA	12	Cisplatin Cyclophosphamide Doxorubicin Prednisone	9	92% RR 3CR 8PR	Shin, Walsh et al. [24]
C-R	Limited stage unresectable	23	Cisplatin Cyclophosphamide Doxorubicin	Not applicable	70% 5 CR 11 PR	Loehrer, Chen et al. [25]

C, chemotherapy; S, surgery; R, radiotherapy; CR, complete response; PR, partial response
*, if incomplete resection

plete tumour resection and also received post-operative radiotherapy. While a median survival rate could not be determined due to the heterogeneous nature of the trials included in the review, five patients had a disease-free survival of more than five years. Of the 11 patients who had a complete resection, all received cisplatin-based chemotherapy.

Several prospective trials have reported a larger percentage of patients proceeding to resection, albeit in smaller series. Rea et al. [22] reported a 100% response rate in 16 patients with stage III or IV thymoma who received neo-adjuvant ADOC chemotherapy. All 16 patients proceeded to surgery, and 11 had a complete resection. The 5 patients for whom complete resection was not possible had adjuvant radiotherapy. This trial reported a median survival of 66 months [22]. Similarly, in another prospective trial, 5 of 6 patients had a compete resection after ADOC [23], and 8 of 12 patients had a complete resection following chemotherapy with cisplatin, cyclophosphamide, doxorubicin and prednisone [24].

An interesting report of 23 patients with advanced thymoma who received chemotherapy and radiotherapy rather than surgery was published by Loehrer et al. in 1997 [25]. Of these 23 patients, 5 complete and 11 partial responses were reported (an overall response rate of 70%), with a median survival of 93 months. These results appear impressive and are competitive with those reported by multi-modality schedules incorporating surgery [25].

This evidence indicates that it is possible to downstage advanced disease, allowing a proportion of patients to have a complete surgical resection. The treatment is tolerable, with the majority of patients completing the planned treatment schedule. From the results of randomized clinical trials it will be possible to define the optimum chemotherapy regimen, the benefit of neo-adjuvant versus adjuvant chemotherapy, and the role of adjuvant radiotherapy.

Identifying At-Risk Groups

Multimodality treatment is warranted in patients at greater risk of relapse or for whom initial surgery is not possible, but is unlikely to improve the cure rates of early stage disease, which is already high with surgery alone. In the past, defining high-risk patients has been complicated by different classification systems. The 1998 WHO histological classification defines six subgroups – A, AB, B1, B2, B3 and C – that carry prognostic importance, as illustrated in a retrospective review of 200 patients with all stages of thymoma treated in a single centre [20]. Stage of disease was found to be the most important determinant of survival, but within stages I and II, the WHO histological subtypes were an independent prognostic marker. Histological subtypes B2, B3 and C had the worst prognosis. When incorporating these different histological subgroups with stage, sub-groups based on risk factors were proposed for patients treated with surgery alone, which enabled the ranking of patients who may benefit from additional systemic treatment [20]. The use of a more refined staging system would be of value in the design of future trials and recommended treatment protocols.

Treatment of Relapsed Disease

Successful treatment of patients who have relapsed after surgery or initial chemotherapy has been reported in cases involving a variety of treatment approaches, from corticosteroids to high dose chemotherapy. The paucity of patient numbers means that data are limited to case reports and small phase II trials. Clearly, treatment options have to be tailored to the needs of individual patients. We report here a summary of the evidence.

For patients with good performance status who have relapsed after initial surgery, chemotherapy using combination regimens can provide palliation of symptoms with relatively few side effects. A more complex problem is the treatment of patients who have already been treated with chemotherapy as a sole modality or as part of a multimodality treatment programme. In general, as in the management of other cancers, re-challenge with the same drug or drug regimen is often unsuccessful.

Second line chemotherapy with different classes of drugs such as the taxanes is being evaluated. Taxanes do not exhibit cross-resistance with carboplatin, cyclophosphamide or etoposide, making them a good second line option. Despite the theoretical advantages of paclitaxel, availability of data on efficacy is limited to a small number of single case reports. Paclitaxel used as a single agent has been reported to provide symptom improvement and possible stabilization of disease in a single heavily pre-treated patient; in a second case report paclitaxel in conjunction with carboplatin was reported to provide palliation in another previously treated patient with thymoma [26–28]. Paclitaxel requires further evaluation in the form of clinical trials.

A more aggressive approach has used high dose chemotherapy with peripheral blood stem cell support. Successful resection of initially inoperable disease has been reported, as have remissions in heavily pre-treated

patients with recurrent disease. This procedure is toxic, causing profound and prolonged myelosuppression. In one study of five patients with relapsed thymoma, progression-free survival ranged from 3.5 to 16.5 months, which is not superior to that achieved with standard combination chemotherapy. In view of the paucity of data regarding this treatment and its considerable toxicity, this approach should only be considered in the context of a clinical trial [29].

Thymic Carcinoma

Thymic carcinoma (WHO histological classification, subgroup C) has a poor prognosis, with invasive disease frequently apparent at presentation, and metastatic disease occurring early in the natural history of the disease. As with thymomas, surgery remains the most important treatment option and complete resection is the most important prognostic factor. However, chemotherapy is used as part of multi-modality treatment approaches and for palliation of advanced disease.

Retrospective review of a case series of 60 patients failed to identify an apparent benefit from chemotherapy [30]. Subsequently, there have been reports of successful palliation with cisplatin-based chemotherapy, albeit in single cases or small case reviews. In a study of seven patients treated with a range of regimens including a modified ADOC regimen and a combination of cisplatin, vinblastine and bleomycin, four obtained a partial response. The response duration ranged from 7 to 15 months [31]. Additional case reports have reported responses to other cisplatin-based combination chemotherapy. A novel approach was the successful treatment with imatinib of a patient with a thymic carcinoma that over-expressed KIT, a frequent finding in thymic carcinomas but not in thymomas [32, 33].

The role of neo-adjuvant and adjuvant chemotherapy remains equally unknown. Cases of thymic carcinoma have been included in prospective trials. Seven cases of thymic carcinoma were among the 15 cases enrolled in a prospective trial of adjuvant chemotherapy reviewed by Hejna et al. [1]. The median survival was 18.4 months, inferior as expected to the patients with thymoma enrolled within this trial.

In summary, while prognosis of thymic carcinoma is poor, palliation is possible and treatment reasonably well tolerated. As with thymoma, the benefit of adjuvant chemotherapy remains to be determined.

The Future

Although surgery remains the treatment of choice, thymoma is a chemosensitive malignancy with high response rates reported to combination chemotherapy.

Cisplatin seems to be an important component of this combination chemotherapy, and provides the best tumour response rates. The use of neo-adjuvant chemotherapy has resulted in downstaging disease, thus increasing the potential for complete resection. The low incidence of thymoma, however, has meant that there has been a paucity of randomised trials and that the optimum systemic therapy in advanced disease is yet to be defined. As more is understood about prognostic factors in thymoma, it should be possible to identify groups of patients for whom chemotherapy either alone or in combination with other treatment modalities may be helpful. Research into the biology of thymomas may identify molecular targets for which novel agents can be developed. With international collaboration in the conduct of randomized trials headway can be made to answer some of these questions. Success in this endeavour would improve the clinical outcome and quality of life of patients with thymoma.

References

1. Hejna M, Haberl I, Raderer M. Nonsurgical management of malignant thymoma. Cancer 1999;85:1871–1884.

2. Talley RW, O'Bryan RM, Gutterman JU, Brownlee RW, McCredie KB. Clinical evaluation of toxic effects of cis-di-amminedichloroplatinum (NSC-119875)–phase I clinical study. Cancer Chemother Rep 1973;57:465–471.

3. Miller AB, Hoogstraten B, Staquet M, Winkler A. Reporting results of cancer treatment. Cancer 1981;47:207–214.

4. Park HS, Shin DM, Lee JS, et al. Thymoma. A retrospective study of 87 cases. Cancer 1994;73:2491–2498.

5. Bonomi PD, Finkelstein D, Aisner S, Ettinger D. EST 2582 phase II trial of cisplatin in metastatic or recurrent thymoma. Am J Clin Oncol 1993;16:342–345.

6. Sofer LF, Gabrilove J, Wolf BS. Effect of ACTH on thymic masses. J Clin Endocrinol Metabol 1952;12:690–696.

7. Hu E, Levine J. Chemotherapy of malignant thymoma. Case report and review of the literature. Cancer 1986;57:1101–1104.

8. Almog C, Pik A, Weisberg D, Herczeg E. Regression of malignant thymoma with metastases after treatment with adrenocortical steroids. Isr J Med Sci 1978;14:476–480.

9. Leinen JG, Wittliff JL, Kostyu JA, Brown RC. Glucocorticoid-binding components in an irradiation-induced thymoma of the C57BL-6J mouse. Cancer Res 1974;34:2779–2783.

10. Tateyama H, Takahashi E, Saito Y, et al. Histopathologic changes of thymoma preoperatively treated with corticosteroids. Virchows Arch 2001;438:238–247.

11. Highley MS, Underhill CR, Parnis FX, et al. Treatment of invasive thymoma with single-agent ifosfamide. J Clin Oncol 1999;17:2737–2744.

12. Berthaud P, Le Chevalier T, Tursz T. Effectiveness of interleukin-2 in invasive lymphoepithelial thymoma. Lancet 1990;335:1590.

13. Gordon MS, Battiato LA, Gonin R, Harrison-Mann BC, Loehrer PJ Sr. A phase II trial of subcutaneously administered recombinant human interleukin-2 in patients with relapsed/refractory thymoma. J Immunother Emphasis Tumor Immunol 1995;18:179–184.

14. Fornasiero A, Daniele O, Ghiotto C, et al. Chemotherapy for invasive thymoma. A 13-year experience. Cancer 1991;68:30–33.

15. Loehrer PJ Sr, Kim K, Aisner SC, et al. Cisplatin plus doxorubicin plus cyclophosphamide in metastatic or recurrent thymoma: final results of an intergroup trial. The Eastern Cooperative Oncology Group, Southwest Oncology Group, and Southeastern Cancer Study Group. J Clin Oncol 1994;12:1164–1168.

16. Loehrer PJ Sr, Jiroutek M, Aisner S, et al. Combined etoposide, ifosfamide, and cisplatin in the treatment of patients with advanced thymoma and thymic carcinoma: an intergroup trial. Cancer 2001;91:2010–2015.

17. Giaccone G, Ardizzoni A, Kirkpatrick A, Clerico M, Sahmoud T, van Zandwijk N. Cisplatin and etoposide combination chemotherapy for locally advanced or metastatic thymoma. A phase II study of the European Organization for Research and Treatment of Cancer Lung Cancer Cooperative Group. J Clin Oncol 1996;14:814–820.

18. Loehrer PJ Sr, Wang W, Johnson DH, Aisner SC, Ettinger DS. Octreotide alone or with prednisone in patients with advanced thymoma and thymic carcinoma: an Eastern Cooperative Oncology Group Phase II Trial. J Clin Oncol 2004;22:293–299.

19. Cowen D, Richaud P, Mornex F, et al. Thymoma: results of a multicentric retrospective series of 149 non-metastatic irradiated patients and review of the literature. FNCLCC trialists. Federation Nationale des Centres de Lutte Contre le Cancer. Radiother Oncol 1995;34:9–16.

20. Chen G, Marx A, Wen-Hu C, et al. New WHO histologic classification predicts prognosis of thymic epithelial tumors: a clinicopathologic study of 200 thymoma cases from China. Cancer 2002;95:420–429.

21. Tomiak EM, Evans WK. The role of chemotherapy in invasive thymoma: a review of the literature and considerations for future clinical trials. Crit Rev Oncol Hematol 1993;15:113–124.

22. Rea F, Sartori F, Loy M, et al. Chemotherapy and operation for invasive thymoma. J Thorac Cardiovasc Surg 1993;106:543–549.

23. Berruti A, Borasio P, Gerbino A, et al. Primary chemotherapy with adriamycin, cisplatin, vincristine and cyclophosphamide in locally advanced thymomas: a single institution experience. Br J Cancer 1999;81:841–845.

24. Shin DM, Walsh GL, Komaki R, et al. A multidisciplinary approach to therapy for unresectable malignant thymoma. Ann Intern Med 1998;129:100–104.

25. Loehrer PJ Sr, Chen M, Kim K, et al. Cisplatin, doxorubicin, and cyclophosphamide plus thoracic radiation therapy for limited-stage unresectable thymoma: an intergroup trial. J Clin Oncol 1997;15:3093–3099.

26. Jan N, Villani GM, Trambert J, Fehmian C, Sood B, Wiernik PH. A novel second line chemotherapy treatment of recurrent thymoma. Med Oncol 1997;14:163–168.

27. Sandler A, Fox S, Meyers T, et al. Paclitaxel plus gallium nitrate and filgrastim in patients with refractory malignancies: a phase I trial. Am J Clin Oncol 1998;21:180–184.

28. Umemura S, Segawa Y, Fujiwara K, et al. A case of recurrent metastatic thymoma showing a marked response to paclitaxel monotherapy. Jpn J Clin Oncol 2002;32:262–265.

29. Hanna N, Gharpure VS, Abonour R, Cornetta K, Loehrer PJ Sr. High-dose carboplatin with etoposide in patients with recurrent thymoma: the Indiana University experience. Bone Marrow Transplant 2001;28:435–438.

30. Suster, S, Rosai J. Thymic carcinoma. A clinicopathologic study of 60 cases. Cancer 1991;67:1025–1032.

31. Kitami A, Suzuki T, Kamio Y, Suzuki S. Chemotherapy of thymic carcinoma: analysis of seven cases and review of the literature. Jpn J Clin Oncol 2001;31:601–604.

32. Pan CC, Chen PC, Chiang H. KIT (CD117) is frequently overexpressed in thymic carcinomas but is absent in thymomas. J Pathol 2004;202:375–381.

33. Strobel P, Hartmann M, Jakob A, et al. Thymic carcinoma with over expression of mutated KIT and the response to imatinib. N Engl J Med 2004;350:2625–2626.

34. Macchiarini P, Chella A, Ducci F, et al. Neoadjuvant chemotherapy, surgery, and postoperative radiation therapy for invasive thymoma. Cancer 1991;68:706–713.

Radiotherapy in the Management of Thymoma

12

Nicholas Bates

Introduction

The modern management of thymoma frequently requires a multi-disciplinary approach. Surgery remains the pivotal treatment modality, and may be the only intervention required in early disease, but radiotherapy has an essential role in the management of more advanced thymomas. Its benefits vary depending on the stage of the disease, but broadly can be divided into three areas, each of which will be reviewed in this chapter:

1. Adjuvant treatment after complete surgical resection of thymoma
2. Part of a multi-modality program for locally advanced unresectable disease
3. Palliation of metastatic thymoma

This chapter will focus on recent data, as others have previously reviewed the field [1–3]. It should be noted, however, that even in recent publications the patients being described may have been treated many years earlier. As there have been major improvements in the quality of radiotherapy, with progress made steadily over many years, reports may include patients who were treated with equipment that today would be regarded as sub-optimal.

Adjuvant Treatment after Complete Surgical Resection of Thymoma

The Role of Adjuvant Radiotherapy in Thymomectomy

Surgical resection can be achieved routinely in stage I and II thymoma, and in a proportion of stage III disease. There are, however, relapses after surgery, and post-operative adjuvant radiotherapy has been used to reduce this risk. Ideally, adjuvant radiotherapy would only be recommended to those patients destined to relapse after surgery. We are, however, a long way from being able to achieve this degree of prognostic precision. Where radiotherapy is used selectively, there will inevitably be some patients who are treated unnecessarily and others who relapse having not received adjuvant treatment. The proportion of people in each group depends upon the level of risk of

recurrence that triggers a recommendation for adjuvant radiotherapy, which varies between centres.

The primary prognostic factors are tumour stage, histological grade and extent of surgical resection. The most commonly used staging system is that described by Masaoka et al. [4], which clearly predicts prognosis. Completeness of excision is not incorporated in this staging system. The WHO histological classification [5] gives additional prognostic information, as was clearly demonstrated by Chen et al. [6]. This large review of 200 thymomas from the Shanghai Chest Hospital achieved a mean follow-up of 15 years. Most relapses will have occurred within this timeframe. A clear difference in outcome was seen according to histological subtype. Type A, AB and B1 tumours had an excellent outcome. In contrast, type B2, B3 and C thymomas did less well, with 5-year survival rates of 75%, 70% and 48%, respectively. The importance of the Masaoka stage was also confirmed, as expected. There is an association between stage and WHO histological grade, such that early stage thymomas are more likely to be types A, AB and B1, while more advanced disease is more likely to be B2, B3 or C. Histological type does, however, give prognostic information independent of stage in stage I and II thymomas, and thus could potentially be used to refine decisions on adjuvant treatment.

There is general, but not universal, agreement that adjuvant radiotherapy is unnecessary in thymomas of Masaoka stage I (complete tumour encapsulation with no microscopic invasion of the capsule). The results from surgery alone in this group are excellent [7] and there is little scope for radiotherapy to produce further improvement. One of the very few randomised trials in thymoma radiotherapy addressed this issue prospectively [8], randomising patients with stage I disease to surgery alone or surgery with post-operative radiotherapy. No relapses occurred during the trial, and there was no demonstrated benefit from radiotherapy. As only 29 patients were randomised, the power of this study to detect a significant difference was limited. The evidence base taken overall, however, indicates that adjuvant radiotherapy should not be used in stage I thymoma. It is possible that this policy should not be followed in special situations. If there has been a breach of the capsule, as a result of rupture at surgery or by an inappropriate pre-operative biopsy, it can be argued that the risk of relapse is higher [9]. Decisions in this situation have to be individualised, as clear evidence is not available.

The role of adjuvant treatment following complete surgical resection of Masaoka stage II disease is less clear. Singhal et al. argue strongly against adjuvant radiotherapy for stage II (and I) thymoma [10]. They reviewed the outcome of 70 patients who had undergone resection for stage I or II thymoma between 1992 and 2002. All had undergone a complete resection. Referral for adjuvant radiotherapy was based on the surgeon's subjective assessment of the risk of recurrence. Three of 30 patients (10%) with stage I disease, and 20 of 40 (50%) with stage II disease underwent radiotherapy. At a median follow-up time of 70.3 months, there had been six intercurrent deaths, but none due to thymoma. Two recurrences had occurred, one each in the irradiated and non-irradiated groups. No significant benefit from radiotherapy was seen.

Similar results have been reported from the Massachusetts General Hospital [11]. In that study, 49 patients with stage II thymoma underwent complete surgical resection. Of them, 14 subsequently received adjuvant radiotherapy and 35 did not. The mean follow-up was 90 months, and only one thymoma recurrence occurred, in a patient who had not received radiotherapy. The recurrence was, however, outside the usual radiotherapy portals.

These results contrast sharply with those of Curran et al. [12]. In a retrospective review, similar in design to those of Singhal and Mangi, 18 patients were identified who had undergone visibly complete resection of a stage II thymoma without post-operative radiotherapy. Six of these suffered a mediastinal relapse and the actuarial 5-year mediastinal relapse rate was 47%. In contrast, these authors found excellent control rates in patients with more advanced loco-regional thymomas that had been treated with radiotherapy. They recommended adjuvant radiotherapy for stage II thymoma. More recently, another study has been reported from Istanbul [13]. In it, 32 patients with completely resected thymomas were reviewed, of whom 24 received post-operative radiotherapy. This had a strong positive influence on progression-free survival, a statistically highly significant finding. In this report, however, patients with resected thymoma were not analysed according to stage, and it is possible that the beneficial effect of radiotherapy was due to the inclusion of patients with resected stage III disease. A similar retrospective study from Ottawa reported on a consecutive cohort of 42 patients with thymoma who underwent surgery [14]. Post-operative radiotherapy was given to most patients with stage II or III disease, and only one death was attributed to thymoma. On the basis of this, the authors recommend adjuvant radiotherapy.

It may be important to consider the histological grade as well as the stage when considering adjuvant radiotherapy. In a retrospective review, Strobel et al. [15] reported the results of 228 patients whose thymomas had been categorised using the WHO classification. They confirmed the findings of Chen et al. [6] that WHO tumour type is a powerful prognostic factor. Consistent with this, good results were obtained for WHO type A, AB and B1 thymomas treated with surgery alone, with three tumour relapses occurring in a group of 76 patients. Prospective randomised studies would be needed, though, to demonstrate conclusively whether histological type should be used to determine adjuvant treatment.

It is not clear why the outcomes reported in these papers differ so markedly. One possibility is that there are systematic differences in the extent of surgery between institutions, but this cannot be determined from the published data. What can be concluded is that the role of adjuvant radiotherapy in completely resected stage II thymoma has not been proven. Further retrospective reviews of outcome are unlikely to give an answer, and this question could best be answered with a multi-centre randomised trial.

In stage III thymoma, complete surgical resection can be achieved in a proportion of cases. However, the relapse rate for this group of patients is higher than for stage II disease and adjuvant radiotherapy; therefore, is of greater potential benefit [16]. It is not possible to select out the low risk patients from this group currently, and it is reasonable to recommend routine adjuvant irradiation in this situation.

Management of Locally Advanced Unresectable Thymoma

It is often not possible to completely resect thymoma that is locally advanced at presentation. This is the case in a variable proportion of Masaoka stage III and virtually all stage IVA disease. Non-invasive investigations do not always predict complete resectability, which ultimately can only be determined at surgery. Many patients in this situation are treated with sub-total resection and post-operative radiotherapy. There may be an advantage, however, to aggressive multi-modality approaches to treatment, using various combinations of chemotherapy, surgery and radiotherapy.

Loehrer et al., in a phase II study, gave two to four cycles of cisplatin, doxorubicin and cyclophosphamide (PAC) chemotherapy as neo-adjuvant treatment [17]. This was followed by radiotherapy to a total dose of 54 Gy to the primary tumour and regional lymph nodes, but no planned surgery. The reported toxicity was mild, and the overall response rate to the combined treatment, based on 23 assessable patients, was 69%. The time to treatment failure was 93.2 months, and the 5-year survival 52.5%.

Shin et al. have reported encouraging results from a multidisciplinary treatment protocol used at the M.D. Anderson Cancer Center in Texas [18]. Patients with unresectable thymoma of Masaoka stage III or IVA were treated with neo-adjuvant chemotherapy using three cycles of cyclophosphamide, doxorubicin, cisplatin and prednisone. Of 12 assessable patients, 3 had a complete response, 8 a partial response and 1 a minor response to chemotherapy. At subsequent surgery in 11 patients, 9 tumours were completely removed and 2 partially resected. Radiotherapy was given to all patients. A dose of 50 Gy was used where there had been complete tumour resection and over 80% necrosis in the operative specimen. With incomplete resection or a lesser degree of necrosis, 60 Gy was used. The median follow-up was fairly short at 43 months, but at that point 10 of 12 patients remained disease-free, and there had been no deaths.

In a recent larger study, Bretti et al. report on the outcome of 63 consecutive cases with stage III and IVA thymoma [19]. In 30 patients primary surgery with radical intent was performed. The remaining 33 received neo-adjuvant treatment, 25 with chemotherapy and 8 with low-dose radiotherapy. Of this group, 12 subsequently underwent successful radical resection. All patients received subsequent radiotherapy. Radical surgery was associated with a longer progression-free survival and overall survival.

Where complete surgical excision is impossible at presentation, the use of neo-adjuvant treatment gives a genuine prospect of down-staging the disease sufficiently to make resection possible. Chemotherapy has several advantages over radiotherapy in this setting. Modern chemotherapy regimens have delivered high response rates, and few patient progress while on treatment. The ability to administer chemotherapy is not restricted if the volume of tumour is large. Radiotherapy, in contrast, carries a real risk of late toxicity if given to a large volume. To get around this, pre-operative radiotherapy has generally been given in a low dose, with a subsequent boost to areas of concern after surgery. This is probably sub-optimal, as split courses of radiotherapy have been shown to be less effective in other clinical situations. A programme of neo-adjuvant chemotherapy, then surgical resection to the greatest extent feasible followed by post-operative radiotherapy, could be usefully investigated in prospective trials.

Radiotherapy Techniques

There has been steady progress in the technology of radiotherapy, which has led to improvements in the quality of treatment. Where patients are recruited into a radiotherapy study over many years, the later entrants are thus likely to have received a superior treatment. In the 1970s, cobalt treatment units were in common use. These machines generate a radiation beam that is of lower energy, and is thus less penetrating, than today's linear accelerators. This lack of penetration resulted in undesirable

variations in absorbed dose across the treated volume. This was a particular problem in patients with a large chest, where the separation between the entry points of the radiation fields is high. This inhomogeneity of dose increased the risk of late toxicity.

Radiotherapy planning, where the volume to be treated is defined, is a fundamental part of the treatment process. Pre-operative diagnostic CT or MRI scans that document the initial extent of disease are useful to ensure that the treated volume is adequate, but this information was not available in the pre-CT era. Radiotherapy planning is now done using CT data generated by a dedicated CT simulator, but many of the patients described in the literature received treatment planned using orthogonal radiographs generated by a conventional simulator. The CT technique is superior in several respects. Accurate characterisation of the tumour bed is easier, although it remains helpful if the surgeon uses clips to mark areas of concern. Normal structures, particularly the lungs, spinal cord and heart, can be accurately defined. This allows the dose they receive to be calculated and presented as a dose-volume histogram, permitting an informed estimate of the risk of toxicity to these normal tissues. Where a risk is unacceptably high, an appropriate adjustment to the radiotherapy plan can be made. Allowance also needs to be made for the increased transmission of radiation through less dense tissue, particularly lung. With CT planning this correction can be made on a pixel-by-pixel basis, an accurate method that reduces variations in the dose of radiotherapy delivered to the tumour.

A further reduction in the risk of radiotherapy-induced toxicity can be achieved by modifying each treatment field to match the shape of the target volume – three-dimensional conformal radiotherapy. This is most easily achieved using multi-leaf collimators, which have come into routine use in recent years, and allow complex field shapes to be swiftly implemented on the treatment unit. Another technique, intensity modulated radiotherapy, can offer advantages in some tumour sites, such as the prostate, but has not yet been demonstrated to be better for treating thymomas.

Volume to be Treated

There is variation between groups in the extent of the volume that is treated with radiotherapy. Particularly in early stage disease, this could be relatively limited, restricted to the tumour bed with margins to allow for microscopic tumour spread and uncertainties in setup. Alternatively, treatment to a larger volume, including the entire mediastinum can be given. Others have advocated irradiating the hemithorax as well as the mediastinum [20]. This wide-field radiotherapy is designed to reduce the risk of tumour recurrence within the pleural cavity, which is otherwise a frequent site of relapse, particularly when pleural invasion is present [21]. Uematsu et al. presented interesting results in the adjuvant setting [20]. Of 43 patients with stage II and III thymomas, 23 received adjuvant radiotherapy to the mediastinum and the entire hemithorax (or in 4 cases the entire thorax), while in 20 only the mediastinum was treated. Patients were not randomised, with the choice of treatment being determined by physician preference. The relapse-free survival was significantly worse in the group receiving mediastinal radiotherapy alone, 66% compared to 100%. There was no significant difference in overall survival. The concern here is with normal tissue morbidity. Although the dose given to the hemithorax field was low, most commonly 15 Gy in 15 daily fractions, there were two cases of severe pulmonary fibrosis in elderly patients, one of which was fatal. As the potential for severe toxicity with these large volumes is significant, more clinical data is needed before this type of treatment can be more widely used.

A similar wide-field technique has been used in advanced thymoma [22]. In this case report, 66 Gy was given to the entire hemithorax of a severely ill patient with advanced thymoma who had not responded to chemotherapy. A very worthwhile clinical response was achieved with tolerable toxicity, but the general applicability of such treatment is unknown. In highly selected patients, who have limited alternative options, it offers potential benefit.

Radiotherapy Dose

A wide range of radiotherapy doses has been recommended for thymoma, and in the absence of randomised trials comparing one dose schedule with another, it is not possible to make evidence-based recommendations. From first principles, however, it is reasonable to use a lower dose in the adjuvant setting, reserving higher doses for macroscopic disease. Typical reported regimens vary from 40 Gy to 60 Gy in the adjuvant setting, and 50 Gy to 70 Gy when treating macroscopic tumour, given in 1.8 to 2 Gy doses. Where various radiotherapy doses have been compared, there has been little evidence of a correlation between dose and tumour control rates [23]. Where radiotherapy is being used for incompletely resected disease, one group has found 50 Gy to be inadequate and has recommended a higher dose [24].

Complications of Thoracic Radiotherapy

Thoracic radiotherapy is generally well tolerated, but has the potential to cause severe or even fatal toxicity. The risk of toxicity increases with the size of volume treated, the total dose delivered and the dose per fraction. Short-term side effects, such as fatigue and radiation oesophagitis, may be troublesome, but resolve within a few weeks of completing treatment. Long-term damage is irrever-

sible, however, and it is this that limits the dose of radiotherapy that can safely be delivered. Late damage to the heart includes accelerated coronary artery disease, pericardial effusions and valve fibrosis, and the oesophagus may be affected with dysmotility and stricture formation. The risk of carcinogenesis from radiation exposure must also be kept in mind, particularly when treating patients whose prognosis is good and where survival for many years can reasonably be anticipated.

The risk of pulmonary toxicity is an important factor limiting the dose of radiotherapy that can be administered to thoracic tumours. Radiotherapy complications are usually classified as either pneumonitis, which occurs during the six months following treatment, or fibrosis, which develops after six months. Both these complications may vary in severity from being asymptomatic, only apparent on chest radiographs, or fatal [25]. The risk of significant pulmonary toxicity is strongly correlated with the volume of lung that is irradiated [26]. This is of particular importance where irradiation of a complete hemithorax is being considered.

Follow-up after Successful Primary Treatment

Thymoma is notorious for its capacity to relapse many years after treatment. For this reason, follow-up should be life-long. Clinical assessment is likely to be abnormal only with advanced disease, so radiological surveillance is required. The evidence base here is very slim, but a suggested policy is to repeat a CT scan of the thorax one, three and seven years after primary treatment. A chest radiograph may be performed at each clinic visit, as despite being insensitive for mediastinal recurrence, it frequently detects pleural disease.

Another reason for undertaking follow-up is to monitor late radiation toxicity. Pulmonary toxicity in particular may cause prolonged symptoms and require supportive management. Oesophageal and cardiac complications may become apparent years after radiotherapy. Personal follow-up of treated patients gives the radiation oncologist an excellent understanding of the resulting toxicity and may suggest ways to refine radiotherapy techniques.

Palliation of Metastatic Thymoma

Unavoidably, some patients will continue to present with thymoma that has already metastasised, or will develop recurrent or metastatic disease after primary treatment. Chemotherapy has an important role in this situation and is discussed elsewhere. Radiotherapy, however, can be of palliative benefit when thymoma deposits are causing significant local symptoms. An example of this is where there has been invasion of the spinal canal, causing spinal cord compression. This use of radiotherapy has not been well documented in the literature, but it is possible to obtain worthwhile improvement in symptoms by the use of relatively low doses of radiotherapy. Simple field arrangements are sufficient in this setting. Doses of 20 Gy in five fractions to 30 Gy in ten fractions give symptomatic improvement with a low risk of significant side effects in most anatomic sites. It is also helpful to manage these patients within a multi-disciplinary team, so that symptom control issues can be addressed appropriately.

Future Directions

The published literature on the use of radiotherapy for thymoma is mostly comprised of single arm non-randomised studies. While these data are valuable, it is necessary to recognise the intrinsic limitations of this type of study. The outcome of non-randomised studies depends on patient selection as well as the efficacy of treatment. To illustrate this, consider the situation where two surgeons, of equal ability, have different criteria for recommending operative management. One applies strict criteria for fitness and advises against surgery in cases where successful resection is in doubt, or where there is significant co-morbidity. The other surgeon is willing to operate on these types of patient. Inevitably the results of surgery will be better for the first surgeon, as patients with an intrinsically poor prognosis have been excluded. The outcome on a population basis, however, will be better for the second surgeon, as more patients will have had access to effective treatment. There are unquantified differences between institutions in the stringency of requirements for trial entry, and this means that results from different centres cannot be directly compared.

Thymoma is a rare disease and even large institutions have difficulty recruiting enough patients to run successful trials. Randomised studies are needed, and co-operative groups are well placed to perform these in a timely fashion. Within the United Kingdom, the National Cancer Research Network has been established to increase recruitment into cancer-related clinical trials. It is hoped that organisations such as this will take on the challenge of organising prospective randomised trials in thymoma.

References

1. Hejna M, Haberl I, Raderer M. Non-surgical management of malignant thymoma. Cancer 1999;85:1871–1884.
2. Dziuba SJ, Curran WJ. The radiotherapeutic management of invasive thymomas. Chest Surg Clin North Am 2001;11:457–466.
3. Johnson SB, Eng TY, Giaccone G, Thomas CR. Thymoma: update for the new millennium. Oncologist 2001;6:239–246.
4. Masaoka A, Monden Y, Nakahara K, Tamioka T. Follow-up study of thymomas with special reference to their clinical stages. Cancer 1981;48:2485–2492.
5. Rosai J, Sobin LH. Histological typing of tumours of the thymus. In: World Health Organization: Histological Typing of Tumours of the Thymus, Springer-Verlag, Berlin, 1999.
6. Chen G, Marx A, Wen-Hu C, et al. New WHO histologic classification predicts prognosis of thymic epithelial tumours. Cancer 2002; 95:420–429.
7. Maggi G, Casadio C, Cavallo A, Cianci R, Molinatti M, Ruffini E. Thymoma: results of 241 operated cases. Ann Thorac Surg 1991;51:152–156.
8. Zhang H, Wang M, Gu X, Zhang D. Postoperative radiotherapy for stage I thymoma: a prospective randomized trial in 29 cases. Chinese Med J 1999;112:136–138.
9. Nagasaka T, Nakashima N, Nunome H. Needle tract implantation of thymoma after transthoracic needle biopsy. J Clin Pathol 1993;46:278–279.
10. Singhal S, Shrager JB, Rosenthal DI, LiVolsi VA, Kaiser LR. Comparison of stages I–II thymoma treated by complete resection with or without adjuvant radiation. Ann Thorac Surg 2003;76:1635–1641.
11. Mangi AA, Wright CD, Allan JS, et al. Adjuvant radiation therapy for stage II thymoma. Ann Thorac Surg 2002;74:1033–1037.
12. Curran WS, Kornstein MJ, Brooks JJ, Turrisi AT. Invasive thymoma: the role of mediastinal irradiation following complete or incomplete surgical resection. J Clin Oncol 1988;6:1722–1727.
13. Eralp Y, Aydiner A, Kizir A, Kaytan E, Oral EN, Topaz E. Resectable thymoma: treatment outcome and prognostic factors in the late adolescent and adult age group. Cancer Invest 2003;21:737–743.
14. Mehran R, Ghosh R, Maziak D, O'Rourke K, Shamji F. Surgical treatment of thymoma. Can J Surg 2002; 45:25–30.
15. Strobel P, Bauer A, Puppe B et al. Tumor recurrence and survival in patients treated for thymomas and thymic squamous cell carcinomas: A retrospective analysis. J Clin Oncol 2004;22:1501–1509.
16. Urgesi A, Monetti U, Rossi G, Ricardi U, Casadio C. Role of radiation therapy in locally advanced thymoma. Radiother Oncol 1990;19:273–280.
17. Loehrer PJ, Chen M, Kim K-M, et al. Cisplatin, doxorubicin and cyclophosphamide plus thoracic radiation therapy for limited-stage unresectable thymoma: an intergroup trial. J Clin Oncol 1997;15:3093–3099.
18. Shin DM, Wlash GL, Komaki R, et al. A multidisciplinary approach to therapy for unresectable malignant thymoma. Ann Intern Med 1998;129:100–104.
19. Bretti S, Berruti A, Loddo C, et al. Multimodal management of stages III–IVA malignant thymoma. Lung Cancer 2004:44;69–77.
20. Uematsu M, Yoshida H, Kondo M, et al. Entire hemithorax irradiation following complete resection in patients with stage II–III invasive thymoma. Int J Radiat Biol Phys 1996;35:357–360.
21. Ogawa K, Toita T, Kakinohana Y, Kamata M, Koja K, Genga K. Postoperative radiation therapy for completely resected invasive thymoma: prognostic value of pleural invasion for intrathoracic control. Jpn J Clin Oncol 1999;29:474–478.
22. Bogart JA, Sagerman RH. High-dose hemithorax irradiation in a patient with recurrent thymoma. Am J Clin Oncol 1999;22:441–445.

23. Ogawa K, Uno T, Toita T et al. Postoperative radiotherapy for patients with completely resected thymoma. Cancer 2002; 94:1405–1413.

24. Mornex F, Resbeut M, Richaud P et al. Radiotherapy and chemotherapy for invasive thymomas: a multicentric retrospective review of 90 cases. Int J Radiat Oncol Biol Phys 1995; 32: 651–659.

25. Jackson MA, Ball DL. Post-operative radiotherapy in invasive thymoma. Radiother Oncol 1991; 21:77–82.

26. Moiseenko, V, Craig T, Bezjak, A, Van Dyk J. Dose-volume analysis of lung complications in the radiation treatment of malignant thymoma: a retrospective review. Radiother Oncol 2003; 67: 265–274.

Overview of Thymic Surgery and Prospective Strategy for Thymic Diseases

13

Kyriakos Anastasiadis and Chandi Ratnatunga

This book has covered the important topics surrounding the thymus gland and its surgery. It has achieved this by recruiting expertise from specialists in different fields, who have provided their own interpretation of the currently available data. Despite originating from one centre, the reader will recognise the variety of opinions among the contributors.

As surgeons, we the authors consider the thymus to be relatively straightforward as a surgical target. Thymectomy can be learnt and performed with relative ease for space-occupying thymic lesions, thymic tumours and myasthenia. Despite this, surgeons have misdirected their energies by trying to devise new and better methods of operating on the thymus rather than focusing on identifying the role and place for surgery in thymic pathology, particularly in myasthenia gravis. This disease does provide the largest cohort of thymic patients in the authors' practices.

One of the aims in writing this book was to draw attention to the need to focus on more important thymic issues. There is a dearth of useful clinical information regarding the management of the disease. Data have been assimilated from a number of series, which have been designed, undertaken and described in a heterogeneous manner. This has left us unable to provide an extensive basis for surgical thymic activity. A clear example of this is in the role of thymectomy in myasthenia gravis. Should we be offering an operation in an era where modern immunosuppression could provide an effective medical thymectomy? Should thymectomy be offered so that immunosuppression could be avoided at all costs? Should thymectomy be offered in late-onset myasthenia? Should it be offered after late presentation or should only in the early stages of clinical presentation? Our dedication to answering some of these questions has led Oxford to enrol itself in the impending multicentre, international trial.

Effort must also be dedicated to mastering the difficult subjects of thymic physiology and immunology. What is the relationship of the central thymus to the circulating T cell immunological forces? What are the precise controlling mechanisms of the thymic neural and humoral pathways that influence thymic function? What is the role of the thymus as an immunological and neuro-endocrine organ?

Thymectomy

The ideal approach for thymectomy for myasthenia gravis is far from settled. Randomised multicentre trials, addressing important issues, are strongly advocated. The Medical Scientific Advisory Board (MSAB) of the Myasthenia Gravis Foundation of America (MGFA) formed an MG clinical classification system (Table 13.1), a grading system of the severity of the disease (Table 13.2), a thymectomy technique classification (Table 13.3), therapy status (Table 13.4) and post-intervention status definition tables (Table 13.5), and a morbidity and mortality classification. These were designed for research purposes so as to achieve more uniformity in future in the recording and reporting of clinical trials and outcomes [1].

Comparing data from trials is also a field of controversy that has to be agreed on with regard to the statistical method to be used. Types of remission analysis techniques that have been used for thymectomy results are: 1) life–table analysis: using the Kaplan–Mayer statistical method; 2) crude remission: the number of remissions/number of thymectomies multiplied by 100% in an unspecified time after the procedure; 3) the hazard rate: remissions per 1,000 patient-months; and 4) the Oosterhuis-Masaoka formula: number of remissions/followed cases multiplied by 100% [2]. Generally, uncorrected crude figures should not be used in comparing data. Life–table analysis may be preferable in the evaluation of remissions when exacerbations are few because it corrects for length of follow-up and patients lost to follow-up. Complete stable remissions, rather than levels of improvement, are the most accurate measure of the effectiveness of thymectomy in the treatment of myasthenia gravis [3]. Randomised trials, meta-analysis and certain statistical methods for comparing data will provide safer conclusions. According to the "Quality Standards Subcommittee of the American Academy of Neurology" report, such trials should include: 1) a prospective patient assembly, 2) thymectomy and non-thymectomy treatment groups with different thymectomy technique arms, 3) randomised assignment to treatment groups or a non-randomised cohort survey with multivariate adjustments for differences in baseline characteristics between groups, 4) standardisation of medical therapies for all patients,

Table 13.1 MGFA MG clinical classification [1]

Class I	Any ocular muscle weakness May have weakness of eye closure All other muscle strength is normal
Class II	Mild weakness affecting other than ocular muscles May also have ocular muscle weakness of any severity
IIa	Predominantly affecting limb, axial muscles, or both May also have lesser involvement of oropharyngeal muscles
IIb	Predominantly affecting oropharyngeal, respiratory muscles, or both May also have lesser or equal involvement of limb, axial muscles, or both
Class III	Moderate weakness affecting other than ocular muscles May also have ocular muscle weakness of any severity
IIIa	Predominantly affecting limb, axial muscles, or both May also have lesser involvement of oropharyngeal muscles
IIIb	Predominantly affecting oropharyngeal, respiratory muscles, or both May also have lesser or equal involvement of limb, axial muscles, or both
Class IV	Severe weakness affecting other than ocular muscles May also have ocular muscle weakness of any severity
IVa	Predominantly affecting limb and/or axial muscles May also have lesser involvement of oropharyngeal muscles
IVb	Predominantly affecting oropharyngeal, respiratory muscles, or both May also have lesser or equal involvement of limb, axial muscles, or both
Class V	Defined by intubation, with or without mechanical ventilation, except when employed during routine post-operative management. The use of a feeding tube without intubation places the patient in class IVb.

and 4) rigidly defined and executed evaluation standards, including masked outcome assessments, systematic reporting of treatment complications, quality of life measures and health care resource usage [4].

With such randomised trials certain conclusions may be extracted about the usefulness, the life-long outcome, the indications, the prognostic factors and the surgical technique of thymectomy for myasthenia gravis. Generally, in the modern era an optimal surgical technique for thymectomy should comprise less invasiveness, maximal radicality [5] and should focus on cosmesis [6]. Use of technology improved the endoscopic techniques with the introduction of robotics in thymic surgery. This new procedure may combine the potential advantages of minimally invasive methods with the efficacy of open procedures [7]. Primary results from this approach are encouraging, even though it needs to be applied in the common practice so as to have certain conclusions about the usefulness and practicality of the technique.

Randomized trials for thymectomy and MG [8]

Since thymectomy has been established as therapy in non-thymomatous MG (based on retrospective, non-randomized studies) and corticosteroids are now being used in-creasingly (either as the sole treatment or in conjunction with thymectomy), a new (multi-center, single-blind, randomized) trial, the MGTX study (Executive Committee: J. Newsom-Davis, GI. Wolfe, HJ. Kaminski, A. Jaretzki, G. Cutter, G. Minisman, R. Conwit and J. Odenkirchen), was designed to investigate the safety while comparing efficacy of prednisone plus extended transsternal thymectomy (ETTX) or no thymectomy (started April 2006, Oxford team was recruited). The results of MGTX study are expected to impact on current clinical practice in the field of MG, either establishing the clinical benefits of ETTX or demonstrating it as an unnecessary procedure in the non-thymomatous MG patients.

A study of biomarkers in MG (which a physician can use to determine how a patient is doing), referred to as BioMG, will be performed as part of MGTX study. BioMG will evaluate three basic biomarkers: 1) genes (called single nucleotide polymorphisms or SNPs), 2) gene expression (the message genes produce), and 3) proteins using patient blood. It is suspected that there are a number of genes that can raise the risk of getting MG. Maybe certain SNPs (which serve as "mileposts" of the human genome) or groups of SNPs will be associated with the diagnosis of MG or possibly predict response to treatment or perhaps even certain side effects. Gene expression patterns evaluate which genes are turned on (ex-

Table 13.2 MGFA quantitative MG score for disease severity [1]

Test Item	None	Mild	Moderate	Severe	Score
Grade	0	1	2	3	
Double vision on lateral gaze right or left (circle one), seconds	61	11–60	1–10	Spontaneous	
Ptosis (upward gaze), seconds	61	11–60	1–10	Spontaneous	
Facial muscles	Normal lid closure	Complete, weak, some resistance	Complete, without resistance	Incomplete	
Swallowing 4 oz water (1/2 cup)	Normal	Minimal coughing or throat clearing	Severe coughing/ choking or nasal regurgitation	Cannot swallow (test not attempted)	
Speech after counting aloud from 1 to 50 (onset of dysarthria)	None at 50	Dysarthria at 30–49	Dysarthria at 10–29	Dysarthria at 9	
Right arm outstretched (90 degrees sitting), seconds	240	90–239	10–89	0–9	
Left arm outstretched (90 degrees sitting), seconds	240	90–239	10–89	0–9	
Vital capacity, % predicted	≥80	65–79	50–64	<50	
Rt-hand grip, kgW					
Men	≥45	15–44	5–14	0–4	
Women	≥30	10–29	5–9	0–4	
Lt-hand grip, kgW					
Men	≥35	15–34	5–14	0–4	
Women	≥25	10–24	5–9	0–4	
Head lifted (45 degrees supine), seconds	120	30–119	1–29	0	
Right leg outstretched (45 degrees supine), seconds	100	31–99	1–30	0	
Left leg outstretched (45 degrees supine), seconds	100	31–99	1–30	0	
				Total QMG score (range, 0–39)	

Table 13.3 MGFA Thymectomy Classification [1]

T-1	Transcervical thymectomy (a) Basic (b) Extended
T-2	Videoscopic thymectomy (a) "Classic" (b) "VATET"
T-3	Transsternal thymectomy (a) Standard (b) Extended
T-4	Transcervical & transsternal thymectomy

Table 13.4 MGFA MG therapy status [1]

NT	No therapy
SPT	Status post-thymectomy (record type of resection)
CH	Cholinesterase inhibitors
PR	Prednisone
IM	Immunosuppression therapy other than prednisone (define)
PE(a)	Plasma exchange therapy, acute (for exacerbations or pre-operatively)
PE(c)	Plasma exchange therapy, chronic (used on a regular basis)
IG(a)	IVIg therapy, acute (for exacerbations or pre-operatively)
IG(c)	IVIg therapy, chronic (used on a regular basis)
OT	Other forms of therapy (define)

Table 13.5 MGFA MG post-intervention status [1]

Complete stable remission (CSR)	The patient has had no symptoms or signs of MG for at least one year and has received no therapy for MG during that time. There is no weakness of any muscle on careful examination by someone skilled in the evaluation of neuromuscular disease. Isolated weakness of eyelid closure is accepted
Pharmacologic remission (PR)	The same criteria as for CSR except that the patient continues to take some form of therapy for MG. Patients taking cholinesterase inhibitors are excluded from this category because their use suggests the presence of weakness
Minimal manifestations (MM)	The patient has no symptoms of functional limitations from MG but has some weakness on examination of some muscles. This class recognizes that some patients who otherwise meet the definition of CSR or PR do have weakness that is only detectable by careful examination
MM-0	The patient has received no MG treatment for at least one year
MM-1	The patient continues to receive some form of immunosuppression but no cholinesterase inhibitors or other symptomatic therapy
MM-2	The patient has received only low-dose cholinesterase inhibitors (< 120 mg pyridostigmine/day) for at least one year
MM-3	The patient has received cholinesterase inhibitors or other symptomatic therapy and some form of immunosuppression during the past year
	Change in Status
Improved (I)	A substantial decrease in pre-treatment clinical manifestations, or a sustained substantial reduction in MG medications as defined in the protocol. In prospective studies, this should be defined as a specific decrease in QMG score
Unchanged (U)	No substantial change in pre-treatment clinical manifestations or reduction in MG medications as defined in the protocol. In prospective studies, this should be defined in terms of a maximum change in QMG score
Worse (W)	A substantial increase in pre-treatment clinical manifestations or a substantial increase in MG medications as defined in the protocol. In prospective studies, this should be defined as a specific increase in QMG score
Exacerbation (E)	Patients who have fulfilled criteria of CSR, PR, or MM but subsequently developed clinical findings greater than permitted by these criteria
Died of MG (D of MG)	Patients who died of MG, of complications of MG therapy, or within 30 days after thymectomy. List the cause (see Morbidity and Mortality table).

pressed) or not. Perhaps, there are gene expression patterns because of their presence or because of their level of activity, can influence how patients respond to treatment. Ultimately, genes direct the expression of proteins, which are the critical building blocks of all cells and tissues of the body. Proteins in the blood of patients will also be tested and correlations made to MG diagnosis and response to treatment during the MGTX study.

The MGFA is also funding a critical ancillary study aiming to produce a classification system (and help to understand how the abnormal thymus is related to the cause of MG) as part of the MGTX study. Linking this study to the MGTX and BioMG is likely to lead to greater insights into MG then could be done otherwise.

Thymus Transplantation

The concept of thymus transplantation for correcting immune deficiencies is an old one, and the first (unsuccessful) attempt was made in the mid 1970s [9]. Since then, organ cultured postnatal thymus has been used in DiGeorge anomaly, AIDS and bone marrow transplants in adults [10]. Although the results from thymus transplantation are as yet unsatisfactory, with properly planned immunosuppression there is some hope for success [10].

Organ transplantation (xenografting) depends on the ability to induce immune tolerance. Concomitant xenografting of thymus and other vascularised organs (simultaneous transplantation of donor/host type thymic epithelium) may induce xenograph tolerance. Host-type thymic epithelial cells may establish self-tolerance, while mixed host/donor thymus grafts may induce T cell xenotolerance and maintain self-tolerance in the recipient [11]. Moreover, the microenvironment of grafted thymus, even if xenogeneic, is able to educate host T cell precursors. This reconstitution of functions, however, does not always induce tolerance to certain auto-antigens and can result in the development of multiple autoimmune lesions to several tissues [12].

Thymus transplantation is comprised of a particular process with elements of solid organ (vascularised) xenografting and cellular infusion (chemotaxis application) therapy. Current techniques utilise culturing T cells in flat sheets and cytokines to drive their growth and differentiation. Because T cells would grow better in an environment that mimicked the three-dimensional structure of the thymus, a matrix used to repair bone (called CellFoam) has been used and seeded with mouse thymus cells and human haematopoietic progenitor cells. This system can mature functional T cells within 14 days. Furthermore, a thymic organoid has been engineered by seeding matrices with murine thymic stroma; co-culture of human bone marrow-derived hematopoietic progenitor cells within this xenogeneic environment also generated mature functional T cells within 14 days [13]. Implantable versions of such thymic organoids (artificial

thymus) that will be able to produce T cells to restore immune deficits are under development. They may also be able to generate populations of T cells to target particular antigens (e.g. tumour antigens) or to induce T cell tolerance to particular antigens (e.g. prevent rejection of a xenograph) [14]. Thymus transplantation and artificial thymus constitute a broad field for research, and may offer a better future to the restoration of acquired or inherited immune deficiencies.

T Cell Utilities

It is much more likely that an extremely rich and diverse, but genetically determined, milieu is present within the thymus, hence the control of intrathymic T lymphocyte maturation and the functional maturation of T cells involving the orchestral interaction of various thymic-specific factors and other molecules during the differentiation process.

Recently, derivatives of thymic hormones, mostly of thymosins, have been detected as products of neoplastically transformed cells and employed in the early diagnosis of neoplasms. In clinical trials, thymic hormones strengthen the effects of immunomodulators in immunodeficiencies, autoimmune diseases and neoplastic malignancies. Combined chemo-immunotherapeutical anti-cancer treatment seems to be more efficacious than chemotherapy alone, and the significant hematopoietic toxicity associated with most chemotherapeutical clinical trials can be reduced significantly by the addition of immunotherapy [15]. Hence, there are perspectives on use of thymic factors in immune deficiency [16].

The thymus is the major primary immune tissue for the production of functional T lymphocytes in humans. Future studies should allow some insight into how to activate specific T cells more effectively for vaccination purposes and how to switch them off to induce tolerance to transplanted tissues [17]. Furthermore, it has been shown that the generation of local T cells also occurs in gut-associated lymphoid tissues (GALT). This suggests that the thymus and GALT have similar functions and that they might be evolutionarily related [18]. If so, this may lead to T cell production from GALT, using them as thymic substitutes to immune system competence.

Alternative Therapies for Thymic Disorders

Immunosuppression with drugs such as prednisone [19], azathioprine [20] and cyclosporine [21] has been successfully used in MG. Experimental immunosuppressive drugs (like mycophenolate mofetil [22]) and techniques (like lymphocytapheresis [23] and immunoadsorption therapy [24]) are under development. Other techniques, such as total body irradiation, have been used in MG, resulting in clinical improvement, probably due to produced lymphopenia and prolonged immunosuppression [25].

Variable immune system secrets are being extensively explored. Future studies may also further clarify how thymic function shapes the repertoire of T cells following stem cell transplant, and demonstrate whether endogenous mediators of thymic function could be selectively applied to regulate post-stem cell transplant thymic function and alloreactivity [26]. Generally, it is not very futuristic to pharmaceutically thymic regeneration, which might become a valuable approach to rejuvenating a depleted peripheral T cell pool [27]. Restoring the immune system may be feasible in future.

References

1. Jaretzki A 3rd, Barohn RJ, Ernstoff RM, et al. Myasthenia gravis: recommendations for clinical research standards. Task Force of the Medical Scientific Advisory Board of the Myasthenia Gravis Foundation of America. Neurology 2000;55:16–23.

2. Jaretzki A III. Thymectomy for myasthenia gravis: analysis of controversies regarding technique and results. Neurology 1997;48(Suppl 5):S52–S63.

3. Jaretzki A 3rd. Outcome after transcervical thymectomy. Ann Thorac Surg 1999;67:592–593.

4. Gronseth GS, Barohn RJ. Practice parameter: thymectomy for autoimmune myasthenia gravis (an evidence-based review). Report of the Quality Standards Subcommittee of the American Academy of Neurology. Neurology 2000;55:7–15.

5. Ruckert JC, Sobel HK, Gohring S, Einhaupl KM, Muller JM. Matched-pair comparison of three different approaches for thymectomy in myasthenia gravis. Surg Endosc 2003;17:711–715.

6. Grandjean JG, Lucchi M, Mariani M. Reversed-T upper mini-sternotomy for extended thymectomy in myasthenic patients. Ann Thorac Surg 2000;70:1423–1425.

7. Ashton RC Jr, McGinnis KM, Connery CP, Swistel DG, Ewing DR, DeRose JJ Jr. Totally endoscopic robotic thymectomy for myasthenia gravis. Ann Thorac Surg 2003;75:569–571.

8. Thymectomy and Myasthenia Gravis. A clinical challenge (MGTX): www.sph.uab.edu/mgtx.

9. Hong R, Santosham M, Schulte-Wissermann H, Horowitz S, Hsu SH, Winkelstein JA. Reconstitution of B nd T lymphocyte function in severe combined immunodeficiency disease following transplantation with thymic epithelium. Lancet 1976;2:1270–1272.

10. Hong R. The thymus. Finally getting some respect. Chest Surg Clin N Am 2001;11:295–310.

11. Xia G, Goebels J, Rutgeerts O, Vandeputte M, Waer M. Transplantation tolerance and autoimmunity after xenogeneic thymus transplantation. J Immunol 2001;166:1843–1854.

12. Morimoto T, Nishigaki-Maki K, Ohno K, et al. Transplantation of xenogeneic embryonic thymus to athymic nude mice induces acquisition of distorted immunity.Transplant Proc 2000;32:956–957.

13. Poznansky MC, Evans RH, Foxall RB, et al. Efficient generation of human T cells from a tissue-engineered thymic organoid. Nat Biotechnol 2000;18:729–734.

14. McCarthy M. Artificial thymus can produce T cells. Lancet 2000;356:48.

15. Bodey B, Bodey B Jr, Siegel SE, Kaiser HE. Review of thymic hormones in cancer diagnosis and treatment. Int J Immunopharmacol 2000;22:261–273.

16. Cunningham-Rundles S, Harbison M, Guirguis S, Valacer D, Chretien PB. New perspectives on use of thymic factors in immune deficiency. Ann N Y Acad Sci 1994;730:71–83.

17. Miller JF. Three decades of T-ology. Thymus 1990;16:131–142.

18. Matsunaga T, Rahman A. In search of the origin of the thymus: the thymus and GALT may be evolutionarily related. Scand J Immunol 2001;53:1–6.

19. Jenkins RB. Treatment of myasthenia gravis with prednisone. Lancet 1972;1:765–767.

20. Mertens HG, Balzereit F, Leipert M. The treatment of severe myasthenia gravis with immunosuppressive agents. Eur Neurol 1969;2:321–329.

21. Tindal RSA, Philips JT, Rollins JA, et al. Preliminary results of a double-blind, randomized, placebo-controlled trial of cyclosporine in myasthenia gravis. N Engl J Med 1987;316:719–724.

22. Schneider C, Gold R, Reiners K, Toyka KV. Mycophenolate mofetil in the therapy of severe myasthenia gravis. Eur Neurol 2001;46:79–82.

23. Furutama D, Nakajima H, Shinoda K, Makino S, Ohsawa N. Lymphocytapheresis in combination with immunosuppressive drugs for refractory myasthenia gravis: two-color flow cytometric analysis of changes in peripheral blood lymphocyte subsets. Eur Neurol. 1995;35(5):270–5.

24. Haas M, Mayr N, Zeitlhofer J, Goldammer A, Derfler K. Long-term treatment of myasthenia gravis with immunoadsorption. J Clin Apheresis 2002;17:84–87.

25. Durelli L, Ferrio MF, Urgesi A, Poccardi G, Ferrero B, Bergamini L. Total body irradiation for myasthenia gravis: a long-term follow-up. Neurology 1993;43:2215–2221.

26. Komanduri KV. Thymic function and allogeneic T cell responses in stem-cell transplantation. Cytotherapy 2002;4:333–342.

27. Berzins SP, Uldrich AP, Sutherland JS, et al. Thymic regeneration: teaching an old immune system new tricks. Trends Mol Med 2002;8:469–476.

Subject Index